The Skidmore-Roth Outline Series:

CRITICAL & HIGH ACUITY

NURSING CARE

2nd Edition

Audree Reynolds, R.N., Ph.D.

Professor
College of Nursing
University of Texas at El Paso
El Paso, Texas

DELMAR

THOMSON LEARNING

Africa • Australia • Canada • Denmark • Japan • Mexico • New Zealand • Philippines
Puerto Rico • Singapore • Spain • United Kingdom • United States

NOTICE TO THE READER

COPYRIGHT © 1995, 1999 Delmar, a division of Thomson Learning, Inc. The Thomson Learning™ is a trademark used herein under license.

Printed in the United States of America
2 3 4 5 6 7 8 9 10 XXX 05 04 03 02 01 00

For more information, contact Delmar, 3 Columbia Circle, PO Box 1-015, Albany, NY 12212-0515; or find us on the World Wide Web at http://www.delmar.com

International Division List

Asia
Thomson Learning
60 Albert Street, #15-01
Albert Complex
Singapore 189969
Tel: 65 336 6411
Fax: 65 336 7411

Japan:
Thomson Learning
Palaceside Building 5F
1-1-1 Hitotsubashi, Chiyoda-ku
Tokyo 100 0003 Japan
Tel: 813 5218 6544
Fax: 813 5218 6551

Australia/New Zealand:
Nelson/Thomson Learning
102 Dodds Street
South Melbourne, Victoria 3205
Australia
Tel: 61 39 685 4111
Fax: 61 39 685 4199

UK/Europe/Middle East
Thomson Learning
Berkshire House
168-173 High Holborn
London
WC1V 7AA United Kingdom
Tel: 44 171 497 1422
Fax: 44 171 497 1426

Latin America:
Thomson Learning
Seneca, 53
Colonia Polanco
11560 Mexico D.F. Mexico
Tel: 525-281-2906
Fax: 525-281-2656

Canada:
Nelson/Thomson Learning
1120 Birchmount Road
Scarborough, Ontario
Canada M1K 5G4
Tel: 416-752-9100
Fax: 416-752-8102

Library of Congress Cataloging-in-Publication Data
Reynolds, Audree
Critical & High Acuity Nursing Care

ISBN: 1-56930-094-1
1. Nursing Handbooks, Manuals.
2. Medical Handbooks, Manuals.

TABLE OF CONTENTS

Preface

The Skidmore-Roth Outline Series: Critical & High Acuity Nursing Care provides the reader with the rationale underlying the nursing care essential for high acuity and critical care conditions. Units on major pathophysiological dysfunction subdivide into sections which address anatomical and physiological overviews, age considerations, key pathophysiological points, interventions to improve function, and examples of common high acuity and critical care conditions. The multiple system involvement which stems from complex and evolving dysfunction contributes to the challenge of this aspect of nursing care.

High acuity and critical care nursing knowledge builds upon a prerequisite understanding of general medical-surgical nursing care and the warning signs of impending complications. High acuity and critical care nursing focuses on relatively unstable clinical situations and multiple system involvement which typically require close monitoring and prompt action to minimize the severity of complications. Persons with high acuity and critical care conditions were traditionally cared for in critical care settings. However, as health care delivery shifts to ambulatory, extended, and home health settings, the principles of high acuity care extend beyond the critical care units to telemetry and skilled-care settings. "High-tech" interventions once seen only in the acute care hospital become common place in nonhospital settings.

This outline provides a concise rationale for high acuity and critical care. The information contained in this text may also supplement other textbooks and references by identifying the essential, "need to know" content as the basis for safe, competent practice. This easy-to-read format serves as a resource for beginning clinicians, new graduates and senior level nursing students caring for individuals with high and multiple system health problems.

In addition to providing the essential content, this text contains several unique learning features. Focused, head-to-toe bedside assessments identify the data usually observed with clinical examples are included. Decision trees provide a schematic of sequences of clinical decision-making related to major clinical manifestations. Patho-flow diagrams depict the sequence of progression of related pathophysiology which may lead to specific complications.

Your comments on the usefulness of the format and content are welcomed as subsequent editions are developed.

Audree Reynolds

Unit 1

Concepts Common to High Acuity and Critical Care Nursing

T his unit addresses concepts common to providing competent nursing care for individuals and their families in high acuity or critical care settings. Most of these conditions begin as relatively simple, stable medical-surgical disorders. Due to a variety of causative factors, the dysfunction progresses to a more complicated situation with multiple body system involvement leading to a variety of potentially life-threatening complications.

Each section in this unit addresses a concept that typically accompanies a high acuity or critical care clinical condition. The common concepts are high-tech care issues, pain management, interventions for disturbed sleep and rest, sensory overload and deprivation, and potential for resuscitation.

Section 1: "HIGH-TECH" CARE ISSUES

1. To practice high acuity or critical care nursing, one must have an in-depth understanding of the body's normal interventions used to restore optimal function. The following issues are often a part of critical and high acuity nursing care:

- Technological advances now provide sophisticated equipment to monitor physiological functions. The care of seriously ill persons frequently equates with "high-tech" care. The array of monitoring equipment at the bedside attests to this premise.

- Care providers become attuned to the equipment and respond to the slightest change emitted from any one of the many pieces of equipment. Each "beep" refers to a specific piece of equipment. Efficient care providers respond appropriately to a slight change in the sound or frequency of each "beep."

- Increasing technology can lead to dehumanization of care. Technology can become more important than the person in the bed, and the focus of care can easily center on curing a symptom and treating a medical diagnosis rather than dealing with the client holistically. For example, a person in bed #1 is often referred to as "the MI in bed #1" rather than "Ms. Rose Jones who has an acute myocardial infarction."

  — Perhaps this response is a self-protective mechanism used by high acuity and critical care providers who experience repeated stress. Depersonalization may protect the care provider temporarily from employment-related stress, but soon care interventions become automatic and impersonal.

  — More optimal approaches for managing employment-related stress foster the use of caring/healing strategies for personalizing care which, in turn, minimize employee "burnout." For suggestions on coping with and effectively adapting to high-stress employment situations, refer to other references on relaxation techniques, debriefing following high-stress episodes, and management approaches for traumatic stress syndrome.

2. Effective high acuity and critical care providers assign equal attention and importance to the technological equipment and the person attached to each machine. The essential fact is that a person is attached to each piece of "high-tech" equipment. All monitoring equipment is merely an extension and sophistication of other assessment techniques. "High-tech" monitoring provides additional data to validate findings   gleaned from less sophisticated techniques.

- One example is an EKG tracing which provides additional data about cardiac function and builds upon physical assessment findings, apical and radial pulse, perfusion data, and specific clinical manifestations. Another example is hemodynamic monitoring which provides additional data about perfusion and builds upon the findings obtained from a cuff blood pressure.

- High acuity and critical care providers sometimes deceive themselves into believing that they heal individuals when, in fact, nurses and physicians do not heal. Rather, they provide an environment in which healing can occur. Healing is a personal and internal process within the person who is ill.

- Humanizing "high tech" nursing care will provide increased opportunities for improved client care. Nursing care techniques and medical therapies will become healing interventions. Holistic nursing care will become integral to high acuity and critical care nursing. Collaboration between each nurse and each physician will focus on the person healing, not merely treating symptoms and curing problems.

Section 2: PAIN MANAGEMENT

Nearly everyone experiences pain. Pain is a personal, private experience often with related observable symptoms. The occurrence and intensity of pain can interfere with rest and maintenance of optimal physiological function. Response to painful situations involves a variety of cultural and personal factors.

Pain accompanies most high acuity and critical care conditions. Effective management of pain facilitates healing and minimizes the development of complications. Reports suggest that effective management of pain during the postoperative period shortens recuperation and that there are fewer complications. In spite of numerous documented findings, some physicians are reluctant to prescribe adequate analgesia for known painful procedures and some nurses are reluctant to administer prescribed analgesics.

1. Descriptive terms relating to pain:

- Localized pain refers to pain confined to a specific site of painful stimuli. An example is incisional pain.

- Projected pain refers to pain along a specific nerve. An example is compression between lumbar vertebrae which causes pain along the sciatic nerve in the leg.

- Radiating pain refers to diffused pain around a specific site which focuses in a defined direction from the original site. An example is chest pain that moves toward the left arm following an acute MI.

- Referred pain refers to pain perceived in an area distant from the site of painful stimuli. An example is intense lower back pain associated with acute pancreatitis.

2. Responses to pain:

- Physiological responses to acute pain include increased or fluctuating blood pressure, increased pulse rate, increased respiratory rate, dilated pupils, and perspiration. Behavioral responses include restlessness, inability to concentrate, apprehension, and distress.

• Physiological responses to chronic pain include normal blood pressure, normal pulse rate, normal respiratory rate, normal pupils, and dry skin. Behavioral responses include immobility or physical inactivity, withdrawal, and despair.

• Use of visual, analog self-rating scales assist care providers in determining the degree of pain (or pain relief) experienced by an individual. This technique is particularly helpful when gaining an understanding of chronic pain or cultural and ethnic factors.

— For example, one person may become very vocal, demonstrative and in apparent acute distress when family members are present. Another person may appear very quiet and stoic. Both persons may perceive and self-rate their pain as "mid-range" and tolerable with little intervention. A care provider may misinterpret the degree of pain experienced by both of these persons and administer too much or too little analgesia.

3. **Pharmacological intervention:**

• Our bodies naturally produce polypeptides, enkephalins and endorphins, which all have an opiate-like analgesic effect. Selected brain tissues produce these substances in response to various factors. The analgesic effect typically alters the painful impulse transmission along CNS pathways. Prolonged strenuous activity, transcutaneous electrical nerve stimulators (TENS), antidepressant therapy, and adequate amounts of serotonin enhance the activity of these substances.

• Non-narcotic analgesics include acetylsalicylic acid (Aspirin) and acetaminophen (Tylenol). Nonsteroidal anti-inflammatory agents (NSAID) manage acute inflammation associated with tissue destruction. Subsequently, pain relief occurs.

— Many non-narcotics are available as over-the-counter preparations. Many persons believe this category of medications is "safe" and ingest them liberally, when in fact, each medication also has an adverse systemic effect. For example, aspirin may produce gastrointestinal irritation and bleeding.

— Narcotics produce potent analgesia, but they have side effects. When administering prescribed narcotics, health care providers worry about the adverse effects such as the possibility of addiction and the effects of drug withdrawal. In fact, addiction infrequently occurs among persons using narcotics for medicinal relief of pain. Undermedication and poor pain management are more likely to occur.

— Examples of narcotics include: morphine sulfate; meperidine (Demerol); codeine; pentazocine (Talwin); oxycodone (Percodan). The management of cancer pain may require long-acting medications, such as levorphanol (Levo-Dromoran). Control-released oral morphine (MS Contin R) may provide sustained pain relief, especially when administered on a regular schedule.

— Certain medications have secondary properties of potentiating the action of narcotics. Their use, in combination with low-dose narcotics, produces desired analgesia. Examples of narcotic potentiators include hydroxyzine (Vistaril) or promethazine (Phenergan).

— Narcotics also produce CNS depression, cardiovascular responses (vasodilation and lowered blood pressure), and gastrointestinal responses (nausea, vomiting, constipation).

— When intense pain occurs, continuous low-dose infusion, particularly of morphine, produces optimal pain relief with minimal CNS depression. Infusion rates are titrated (adjusted) to meet individual needs.

• Epidural analgesia refers to the instillation of a pain-blocking agent into the epidural space. Pain relief occurs at the level of and below the injection site.

• Patient-controlled analgesia (PCA) is method for managing acute pain. When PCA is used, individual satisfaction is high, pain relief is effective, and daily narcotic consumption decreases. An infusion pump delivers a desired amount via an intravenous or subcutaneous catheter. The use of a locked drug reservoir system, which delivers only a pre-determined amount of drug within a specified interval, minimizes inadvertent overdose.

4. Physical measures for analgesia:

• Physical measures relieve contributing factors and alter the perception of pain. A hand firmly placed on or around the painful area minimizes localized pain. Massage relaxes tense muscles which often accompany bone, muscle, and joint pain. Application of local heat includes diathermy, ultrasound, melted paraffin, Hubbard tank, and hot tub.

— A comfortable environment with clean, unwrinkled sheets and dimmed lighting enhances physical relaxation. Presence of friends and family members and soothing music are additional distractors which may alter the perception of pain.

— Audio relaxation tapes used in combination with physical measures assist in progressive relaxation of body muscles. This approach enhances the effectiveness of other measures.

- Transcutaneous electrical nerve stimulation (TENS) manages acute and chronic pain through the use of a battery-operated device which intermittently delivers small electrical currents to the skin and underlying tissues. The person perceives a prickly, pins and needles sensation with the delivery of the currents.

- Acupressure/acupuncture involves the application of pressure or insertion of tiny needles into the subcutaneous tissue at specific anatomical locations (meridians). Altered impulse transmissions along nerve pathways produce relief of pain in many situations. Many persons believe that this treatment modality cures some illnesses.

- Biofeedback involves the self-monitoring of various physiological responses by a small electronic sensor. Galvanic skin response and skin temperature reflect changes in peripheral blood flow, heart rate, and blood pressure. The combination of biofeedback and other noninvasive measures assist the individual in gaining self-control over systemic responses in the management of chronic pain.

- Imagery is a form of distraction in which the person mentally visualizes pleasant feelings, sensations or events at the onset of pain. A facilitator assists the person in sustaining a sequence of thoughts and the desired mental image.

- Hypnosis refers to an altered state of consciousness in which the altered perceptions of selected conditions (pain) occur without affecting the person's contact with reality or his or her understanding of what is happening. This technique is helpful in the management of chronic pain.

- Therapeutic touch involves the placing of a provider's hands on, or close to, the painful site. A slow, rhythmic movement of the hands over and away from the site accompanies a soothing sensation and a decrease in the intensity of the pain. Positive response to this noninvasive technique includes a decrease in perceived pain, an increase in the individual's sense of well-being, and decrease in blood pressure and pulse rate.

5. Surgical intervention:

- Operative procedures interrupt the pain pathways when the pain is intractable or severely debilitating. Nerve blocks involve the destruction of a nerve root with the injection of a chemical agent such as phenol or alcohol. A rhizotomy, chordotomy and sympathectomy surgically disrupt impulse transmission along sensory pathways thereby decreasing the perception of pain.

Section 3: DISTURBED SLEEP AND REST

Sleep refers to a naturally occurring state of relative unconsciousness during which the cerebrum rests and selected systemic physiological functions occur. External and sometimes internal stimuli arouse a person from this state. Sleep is a physiological restorative state.

1. Physiology of sleep:

- The sleep-wake cycle is one of the circadian rhythms of the body. The pattern approximates the 24-hour cycle of lightness and darkness.

- Arousal from a sleep state originates in the reticular activating system (RAS) located in the brain stem. Dysfunction within this portion of the brain results in abnormal sleep patterns or an unconscious, sleep-like state.

- Various hormonal changes alter neurotransmission and accompany sleep states. Certain diseases, hormonal disturbances, and medications alter neurotransmission affecting not only sleep but also sensory processes, mood, and cognition.

2. Stages of sleep:

- The sleep cycle can be divided into two categories: REM (rapid eye movement) and NREM (non-rapid eye movement). In adults, each sleep cycle follows a sequence of REM and a series of progressively deeper NREM stages. Each cycle lasts about 90 minutes. Most persons move through an orderly sequence of progressively deeper sleep with a return to lighter sleep. Typically, 4-5 cycles occur during a nighttime sleep period.

  — During REM sleep, persons exhibit characteristic lateral eye movements that are observable through closed eyelids. Erratic respirations, changes in heart rate, and decreased temperature occur. Respiratory activity is primarily diaphragmatic with minimal use of accessory muscles. Response to hypoxia and hypercapnia decreases. Dreams during REM sleep are vivid, story-like, emotional, and often bizarre. During stage 1 and 2, REM sleep is "light" sleep from which a person can be easily aroused. Physiological activities become slow and stable.

  — Stages 3 and 4, NREM sleep, refer to slow wave sleep (SWS) during which characteristic brain waves are low-frequency and high-voltage delta waves. The characteristic waves of SWS differentiate sleep from coma. Also, with SWS, oxygen consumption by muscle tissue decreases. Respirations become slow and even. Dreams during NREM are ruminations of recent events with little story value.

3. Need for sleep:

- During a sleep state, the action of the parasympathetic nervous system increases. Sleep restores energy to the brain and central nervous system. This process resembles resetting or recalibrating a machine to a baseline.

- During sleep, the body actively repairs and restores itself. Restorative, reparative and growth processes occur during slow-wave sleep which accompany the deeper sleep stages (3 and 4). Synthesis of brain activities associated with learning, reasoning and emotional adjustment occur during early sleep or REM sleep.

- Activation of the parasympathetic nervous system occurs during sleep. Some of these activities include: release of growth hormone, increase in digestion and absorption of ingested nutrients, tissue generation and repair, healing and regeneration, synthesis of hormones and enzymes, and synthesis of immunoglobulins.

  — Without adequate amounts of REM and NREM sleep, persons with high acuity and critical care conditions will experience impaired healing and prolonged recovery.

4. Sleep disturbances and body system dysfunction:

- Insomnia and fragmented sleep frequently occur with Parkinson's disease, a disorder related to imbalances in neurotransmission.

- Frequent wakening and agitation accompany Alzheimer's disease.

- Head injuries produce a wide variety of disturbances in sleep patterns that may last for several weeks or months. A sleep-like state of unconsciousness may occur with specific infratentorial lesions. During these states, some sensory pathways are intact and function within normal parameters.

  — For example, hearing often remains intact even when no apparent response is observable. Conversations at the bedside should include the person as if normal hearing is present. Address the person with respect and avoid informal names, such as "gramps" or "sweetie." Conduct discussions about poor prognosis, other patients, or personal topics beyond the patient's hearing range.

- Diabetes mellitus type I may produce hypoglycemic episodes during the night. Subtle signs include nightmares and early morning headaches. More typical signs of hypoglycemia include sweating, palpitations, hunger, and anxiety.

- Nocturnal asthmatic attacks, which contribute to frequent wakening, are common in cases of poorly managed asthma. Oxygen saturation may fall, especially during REM sleep, resulting in dysrhythmias. Sleep apnea may occur.

- Persons with hypertension are at risk for episodes of obstructive sleep apnea. An association exists among snoring, apneic episodes, and hypertension.

- Persons with severe congestive heart failure often experience periodic breathing that resembles Cheyne-Stokes pattern during stage 1 and 2. Frequent arousal and reduced total sleep time result.

- Variability in heart and respiratory rates is an underlying factor contributing to nocturnal angina. Persons deprived of sleep during a stay in critical care may experience REM rebound following transfer to another care unit. Increased cardiac activity occurs during REM sleep and may produce dysrhythmias.

- Sleep deprivation and erratic sleep patterns reduce the seizure threshold which may trigger seizure activity.

Example of a philosophy statement regarding sleep and rest used in one ICU/CCU:

It is understood that, due to the inherent qualities of the intensive care environment, sleep disruption and/or deprivation can be a serious complication for patients who require this form of nursing care.

Recognizing the potentially serious consequences of sleep deprivation to our patients, (fragmentation and psychosis as well as prolonged hospitalization), we, as nursing care providers, will strive to promote optimum quantity and quality of sleep with the following measures:

I. Information about the patient's usual sleep activity will be incorporated into the nursing care plan and followed as closely as is feasible.

II. When planning care, procedures will be scheduled to protect, or at least minimally disrupt, those hours that are usually spent in uninterrupted sleep.

III. The nursing care plan will reflect cognizance of the fact that the sleep cycle is 90 minutes in length, and group activities will be scheduled so that protected times of undisturbed sleep will be of 90-minute intervals.

IV. Nursing staff must be continually aware of their own and their colleagues' contributions to noise and take responsibility for control of the environment, especially in regard to lights and noise.

V. The monitoring of vital signs will be a judgment call of the nurse caring for the patient and will be based on that nurse's familiarity of the patient's stability, the availability of noninvasive monitoring devices and the amount of sleep disruption that has occurred or will occur for that patient.

American Heart Association, Cardiovascular Nursing, Vol. 19. September-October 1983.

Section 4: SENSORY OVERLOAD AND DEPRIVATION

With optimal sensory processing, an individual initiates and maintains contact and interaction with others and one's environment. Normally, a person adapts to the frequency and intensity of input stimulation. When an acute illness occurs, a disruption in the balance between familiar input and adaptive responses develops. Sensory input often becomes excessive; the result is overload or inadequate, meaningless stimulation. Sensory overload may lead to deprivation of appropriate and meaningful input. Behavioral and systemic manifestations appear when prolonged imbalance exists.

1. **Clinical manifestations of sensory imbalance:**

   - Physical changes include: drowsiness; yawning; prolonged and frequent sleep periods; altered motor coordination

   - Perceptual changes include: visual and auditory distortions; unusual body sensations (tingling, numbness)

   - Cognitive changes include: poor concentration; bizarre ideas; impaired memory; confusion; disorientation

   - Emotional changes include: anxiety; depression; crying; fear; mood swings; anger

2. **Sensory deprivation** refers to the reduction in variety and intensity of meaningful sensory input. One example of sensory deprivation occurs when a physical condition causes a person not to recognize and interpret meaningful stimuli from the environment. In this situation, the stimuli are appropriate but not perceived as meaningful by the individual. Another example occurs when health care providers focus their attention more on the "high-tech" equipment at the bedside rather than interaction with the individual.

   - Normal physiological changes that occur among the elderly may accentuate the sensory deprivation. Total darkness accompanied by impaired eyesight often precipitates increased alertness and may lead to confusion. Sounds are often distorted and low tones are often muffled which produces a startled response to sudden high-frequency sounds.

— Immobility and sensory loss increase an individual's feeling of separation from his or her environment. Impaired hearing and misinterpretation of
normal conversation often occurs, especially in a
bedside environment with monitoring equipment
and alarms. In this situation, input stimulation
becomes inappropriate and meaningless.

— The presence of pain often accentuates altered sensory input. A distortion of time frequently occurs.
For example, when experiencing pain, an interval
of five minutes is typically perceived as consider-
ably longer. A feeling of misunderstanding, isolation and loneliness increases.

• Interventions to minimize sensory deprivation
include:

— Protection of the eyes from injury and strain is
accomplished by providing adequate light during
periods when the client is awake and dimmed
bedside lighting for rest and sleep to provide for
periods of stimulation and rest. Avoiding overbed
lighting which may shine directly into the person's
eyes will decrease inappropriate stimulation.

— Self-introduction by the care provider when
approaching the bedside decreases a startle
response and promotes trust. Providing a simple
statement about place and time promotes orientation. A bedside clock and calendar facilitate the
comprehension of the passage of time.

— Family members who stay with the person and
engage in conversation about topics of interest to
the person promote a trusting environment. Audio
tapes with earphones of family conversations also
provide meaningful stimulation.

— When possible, moving the person out of his or
her bed and, if reasonable, away from the imme-

diate bedside provides new sensory input. Sitting in a chair in the hallway or visitor waiting area provides the individual with a wealth of new and different stimuli.

— The typical hospital environment perpetuates isolation and diminished frequency of meaningful stimulation. The walls of a hospital are typically pale and often lack pictures. Critical care units often do not have windows or natural sunlight to provide day/night cues. Hospital linens and uniforms of personnel are monotone and color coded by department. Confinement to bedrest and immediate bedside limits a hospitalized person's personal space. Restricted visiting hours control the contact with significant others, and, thereby, limit personalized and meaningful stimulation.

3. **Sensory overload** refers to an increase in environmental stimuli which are often multisensory. Bombardment results in meaningless input. The frequency or intensity of stimulation occurs faster than the ability of an individual to appropriately respond. Typically, the individual remains in a prolonged state of alertness and altered sleep patterns. Sleep deprivation contributes to sensory overload.

   • One example of sensory overload occurs when bedside lighting remains constant for hours. Bright lights often remain on 24 hours each day in critical care units. Dimming the lights when physical contact with the person is not needed encourages rest periods.

   • Another example of sensory overload results from the bombardment of sounds from bedside equipment and monitoring devices. Care providers become accustomed to these sounds which are unfamiliar to an acutely ill person and his or her family. Adjustment of the volume of alarms is sometimes possible. In relatively stable situations, a decrease in the intensity of bedside alarms is often feasible.

Centrally located monitoring alarms remain unchanged. Thus, continuous monitoring assesses physiological status and a quieter bedside environment is achieved.

— A major source of noise in a critical care unit is conversation among the care providers. Loud verbal dialogue outside the room about unrelated topics produces unnecessary stimulation. Housekeeping activities and movement of equipment compound the noise level and sensory overload. Other sources of nonessential noise include radios and television. Care providers often do not realize that they are producing nonessential stimulation.

• When bedside monitoring and equipment provide excess noise stimulation, the use of audiotapes with earphones provides soothing sounds which often block out the "white" noise generated by the surroundings. Beneficial effects of this strategy include a decrease in and stabilization of blood pressure and pulse rate.

Section 5: POTENTIAL FOR RESUSCITATION

Persons experiencing high acuity and critical care conditions are at high risk for developing sudden and severe changes in their physiological functioning. Knowing an individual's baseline and trends in physiological changes alerts the bedside nurse to a potential and evolving deteriorating state. Often these changes are reversible, but sometimes the status continues to deteriorate, resulting in a cardiopulmonary arrest.

1. Warning signs of impending arrest:

• As a general guideline, adults typically exhibit deteriorating changes in circulation or perfusion before exhibiting changes in their respiratory status. Thus, adults are more likely to experience deteriorating circulatory status which, if undetected and untreated, leads to cardiac arrest. Respiratory arrest follows cardiac arrest with this age group.

— For adults without cardiac or hemodynamic monitoring, warning signs relate to decreasing perfusion of oxygenated blood to the heart muscle and brain. Increasing cardiac ischemia and chest pain develop. Cardiac monitoring reveals an onset of or increase in dysrhythmias—particularly PAC or PVC. Progressive bradycardia may be another warning sign of impaired myocardial effectiveness.

— Increasing mental confusion, restlessness, and anxiety accompany decreasing cerebral oxygenation and perfusion.

• As a general guideline, infants and children exhibit signs of deteriorating respiratory status before impaired circulatory function. Thus, infants and children are more likely to experience a respiratory arrest with few signs of evolving respiratory failure. Unless an underlying cardiac problem is present, infants and children rarely exhibit PAC's or PVC's in an impending arrest situation. A cardiac arrest follows a respiratory arrest with this age group.

— Therefore, close assessment of the adequacy of respiratory function is essential. Prompt intervention to correct a deteriorating status is the appropriate action. Thus, avoiding a respiratory arrest is often possible.

Resuscitation

1. **Cardiopulmonary arrest** is the most serious of all medical and surgical emergencies. Cessation of breathing and circulation is related to an arrest and signifies clinical death. Unless appropriate action is initiated within 4-6 minutes, biological death occurs. If delay in restor-

ing cardiac and pulmonary function is longer than 6 minutes, irreversible brain damage occurs.

- Immediate and effective cardiopulmonary resuscitation (CPR) administered to a victim of sudden death often prevents biological death or irreversible brain damage.

- Cardiopulmonary resuscitation (CPR) involves basic life support (BLS) and advanced cardiac life support (ACLS).

2. **Basic life support (BLS)** involves the recognition and immediate treatment of an airway obstruction or cessation of cardiac or respiratory activity. Appropriate implementation of CPR techniques restores cardiac and respiratory function.

- CPR consists of establishing an airway and administering breathing and circulation.

3. **Advanced cardiac life support (ACLS),** provided by highly trained personnel who use special equipment and medications, restores optimal cardiac and respiratory function. These techniques support BLS measures.

- Adjuncts to airway and breathing include oxygen administration, placement of artificial airway, endotracheal intubation, bagging devices, mechanical ventilation, and endotracheal suctioning.

- Adjuncts to artificial circulation include the continuation of manual chest compressions, automatic chest compression, use of antishock trousers, intra-aortic balloon pump, internal cardiac compression, and automatic external defibrillators.

    — Continuous cardiac monitoring provides data on the effectiveness of cardiac activity and the prompt detection of dysrhythmias. Defibrillation of an ineffective electrical activity of the ventricle may reverse a potentially lethal dysrhythmia.

- Prompt establishment of intravenous access is crucial for the administration of fluids and specific medications. It is crucial to establish this "lifeline" access early in the resuscitation effort as intense peripheral vasoconstriction occurs.

  — Medications administered during an arrest have profound systemic effects in restoring desired cardiac function. Specific algorithms delineate the sequence of medication administration and interventions for each cardiac dysrhythmia.

4. Terminating CPR:

- Resuscitation efforts continue until one of the following events occurs:

  — Restoration of effective circulation and ventilation is accomplished.

  — A physician (or physician's designate) declares the resuscitation effort futile. Effective circulation and ventilation are not restored in spite of appropriate treatment.

  — Exhaustion of resuscitation personnel occurs.

Resuscitation Outcomes

There are three possible outcomes from a resuscitation episode:

- Restoration of physiological function, or a near death experience

- No effective restoration of cardiac or ventilatory activity, or biological death

- Restoration of cardiac and ventilatory activity with irreversible brain damage (brain death)

1. Near Death Experiences (NDE):

- Survivors of cardiopulmonary arrest describe several common experiences and perceptions. During clinical death, persons describe a feeling of comfort, absence of pain, and relaxation. They are aware that they have died. Many persons experience a separation from their bodies. They sense that they are in the corner or above the resuscitation activities watching the process. Some persons describe a sense of frustration that they are unable to communicate with or provide reassurance to the resuscitation personnel.

- Some persons describe movement along a dark tunnel that has an unbelievably bright, warm light at the end, a beautiful meadow, or peaceful place. After successful resuscitation, some persons experience a sense of movement back to the bedside and return of wholeness, or unity, with their physical bodies.

- Not all persons recall these experiences following a resuscitation effort. Some persons want to talk about their perceptions; others do not. Some persons relive their NDE in dreams. Some persons are very uneasy about their experience and feel a sense of frustration, loneliness, or helplessness. Others describe a feeling of peace and acceptance of their own mortality.

- Most persons are reluctant to discuss their experiences and perceptions for fear of being labeled as "crazy." Establishing a caring, trusting, and nonjudgmental climate and initiating the topic often encourages discussion. Statements similar to the following ones may be helpful to some persons who have experienced NDE. "Some persons who experience a similar successful resuscitation recall some unusual feelings. If you have any unusual feelings or memories and would like to talk about them, I'm here to listen."

2. Biological Death:

- Biological death occurs when there is no response to resuscitative efforts. The person is pronounced dead, and the family is notified.

- Some accounts in the professional literature discuss the benefits of the family being present during a code/resuscitation effort. For the experience to be a positive one, a health care provider needs to coach and support the family member through the experience. On the other hand, the presence of the family often is difficult for the health care providers. A code or resuscitation effort does not always proceed in a smooth sequence as typically depicted on television. The risk for misinterpretation of events by an uninformed family member evokes feelings of distrust and skepticism among providers who have not experienced the positive outcomes.

  — Each clinical situation requires careful assessment and decision making to potentially provide the most benefit to family members and providers. Typically, little time is available and there are too few providers to accomplish both an optimal experience for stress-filled family members and the execution of a successful resuscitation.

- In situations in which there was no response to resuscitative efforts, an evaluation for the procurement of non-heartbeating tissue donation may be done. Types of "non-heartbeating" organs and tissues include corneas, skin, bone, ligaments.

- Although the criteria for "non-heartbeating" (cardiac death) donation may vary with institutions, generally guidelines include:

  — General age limits: newborn to no upper age limit

  — Procurement occurs within 24-48 hours of declaration of biological death. Donated tissue are often preserved until transplantation.

3. Brain Death:

Brain death following a resuscitation effort refers to the restoration of cardiac activity without restoration of cerebral activity. This unfortunate situation may also occur following sudden cerebral trauma, such as severe head injury, ruptured cerebral aneurysm, or gunshot to the head.

- Occasionally, despite vigorous and aggressive therapy, a person with serious intracranial disease or trauma develops severe intracranial pressure with irreversible cerebral ischemia. Cessation of cerebral function occurs. With sophisticated cardiopulmonary technology, it is possible to maintain a body's cardiac and gas exchange activities without achieving cerebral activity. In these situations, the discontinuation or withdrawal of technological, mechanical support is considered.

  — It is important to clarify the difference between coma and brain death. Coma is an unresponsive state with evidence of cerebral activity. Brain death is also an unresponsive state, but there is no cerebral activity. Brain death should not be confused with coma; these terms are not interchangeable.

  — A person who is brain dead has lost the ability to hear or to feel pain. The person looks as if he or she is peacefully sleeping. Skin color is usually good because the ventilator is providing optimal gas exchange. The chest moves regularly and smoothly because the ventilator is delivering all respiratory activity.

  — Without cerebral activity, there is no possibility of regaining consciousness or vital functions of breathing and heartbeating. This is difficult for family members to comprehend because reports of "miraculous recovery from death" appear in the tabloids. Such reported incidents of recovery are from deep or prolonged coma rather than from brain death.

- Specific criteria must be met before withdrawal of any technological support occurs. The client must be normothermic and not influenced by any CNS depressant medication or illicit drugs. Physiological criteria include:

  — No evidence of spontaneous respiratory activity

  — Absence of response to the most painful stimuli

  — Absence of cephalic reflexes

  — Minimum of 2 consecutive isoelectric ("flat") EEG that are at least 24 hours apart

  — Absence of cerebral circulation as demonstrated on cerebral angiography (the most accurate indicator of brain death)

- After the decision to terminate technological support equipment is made, restoring the bedside area and person to a pre-crisis atmosphere is important for the family. Bathing the person and combing the hair provides a peaceful, calm appearance. Invasive tubing and equipment are removed from the person and from the immediate bedside area. The bedside and person are neat and clean. The family is encouraged to be with the person as long as they desire. Supportive staff including a nurse counselor and/or clergy are available for the family. Bedside lighting is dimmed because skin color becomes dusky and often mottled as perfusion diminishes.

  — Following the discontinuation of technological support, the heart often continues to beat in a reflex or agonal pattern for several minutes before total cessation occurs. Often, the bedside cardiac monitor screen is turned off, but the central monitoring remains functioning for documenting the cessation of cardiac activity. The waiting period between the time that equipment is terminated and death is pronounced is often stressful for staff and family.

— Debriefing following this event is important for the family and staff. Often, staff members do not take time to deal with their feelings because there is always so much to be done for other persons in a critical care or emergency setting. Debriefing the staff who cared for this person restores emotional energy and coping strategies. Without addressing these events, emotions may accumulate and contribute to "burnout" with clinical manifestations resembling post-traumatic stress syndrome.

- Situations involving brain death are evaluated for the victim's possible eligibility of being a "heartbeating" donor. The bedside nurse is often in a pivotal position of recognizing a potential donor and coordinating communication among the key providers of care and the family. Institutional policy provides guidelines and procedures for referral and consultation with organ procurement agencies.

  — Types of organs included as "heartbeating" are the heart, lungs, pancreas, kidneys, and liver.

  — It is important to identify a potential candidate before declaration of biological death. Families require time to adjust and to cope with a situation of inevitable death. Arriving at a decision for organ donation requires consistent and compassionate communication among care providers, the family, and, preferably, experienced counselors. Supportive counseling is beneficial for the family's decision either to become or not to become a donor.

- Although the criteria for "heartbeating" organ donation may vary with institutions, the general guidelines include:

  — No history of pathology, infection, or substance abuse of the potential donor organ/tissue. Optimal physiological function of the potential donor organ (related laboratory values are all within normal range).

— Negative laboratory testing for hepatitis and HIV.

— General age limits: newborn to 60 years for kidney, liver, or bone marrow; newborn to 40 for heart, lung, or pancreas.

— Transplantation occurs within a few hours of procurement.

• During the period of decision contemplation, specific screening and care interventions are required. Laboratory testing includes physiological compatibility between the donor and recipient cell type and assessment of undetected pathology such as hepatitis and HIV.

— Preservation of the potential "heartbeating" organs requires the meticulous implementation of specific protocols to preserve optimal physiological function of the donor organs and tissues.

• Once the decision to make the client a donor is made, time becomes valuable, and the activity level heightens. Arrangements for "heartbeating" organ procurement and transplantation requires extensive coordination. Often, these arrangements involve physicians and a team of providers located at two or more hospitals in different cities.

• Throughout this process, family members require compassionate, caring support. They have the right to change their decision any time before the procurement procedure begins in the operating room. Most families choose to leave the unit and the hospital after making their decision to donate. Other families choose to stay near the unit or at the bedside until the donor leaves the unit for the procurement procedure.

• When the donor leaves the unit for the procurement

procedure, the staff members frequently experience a variety of emotional states. Some experience feelings of joy and satisfaction that something good came from an unfortunate and often tragic event. Yet, a tremendous feeling of loss and "let-down" occurs because the activity is suddenly over. Staff benefit from debriefing sessions led by experienced personnel and from having an opportunity to express their grief and loss.

Unit 2

Care of Individuals with High Acuity Respiratory Conditions

This unit addresses a variety of high acuity respiratory conditions associated with varying degrees of impaired gas exchange. Persons with these conditions have traditionally been cared for in critical care units. However, as the trends in health care delivery shifts to ambulatory, extended, and home care settings, the principles of high acuity nursing care and related nursing interventions will extend beyond the walls of the traditional acute care hospital.

An understanding of general medical-surgical nursing is the basis for the information presented in this unit. The prerequisite understanding includes normal anatomical considerations, mechanics of breathing and assessment of uncomplicated respiratory status. The extension, elaboration, and refinement of these concepts provide the foundation for nursing care of high acuity respiratory conditions.

Section 1: REVIEW & OVERVIEW

While this unit focuses on pulmonary dysfunction, there is a close interrelationship between the effective functioning of the lungs and the heart. The concept of cardiopulmonary functioning therefore is commonly accepted. Dysfunction of one system may lead to the dysfunction of the other. The resulting alteration in perfusion and hypoxemia may contribute to dysfunction of other organs and possibly lead to multisystem organ failure (MSOF). Prompt recognition of changes in respiratory function and the initiation of appropriate interventions can minimize the severity of this cascade of pathophysiological events.

Anatomical Review

The pulmonary system is located within the thorax and includes two lungs, conducting airways and pulmonary blood vessels. Two layers of serous membrane or pleura surround the lungs. Ciliated mucosa line the upper airways and protect the lower airways from the entrance of foreign bodies and microorganisms. Gas exchange occurs in the 300 million alveoli which comprise adult lung tissue. Surfactant coats each alveolus to maintain expansion and optimal gas exchange.

Age Variation:

As the airway diameter is smaller in infants and children, relatively small amounts of mucous accumulation, constriction or edema can impair air flow.

- The shape of the infant and toddler chest is more round and is very compliant as compared to an adult chest.

Mechanics of Breathing Review

The physiological actions of the pulmonary system include ventilation (breathing) and gas exchange. Oxygen and carbon dioxide move across capillary membranes at the alveolar level. An adequate functioning heart, blood vessels and red blood cells transport these gases throughout the body. Perfusion refers to this process of transportation and cardiopulmonary function refers to the integrated relationship between cardiac, pulmonary, and hemopoietic body systems.

1. **Ventilation (breathing)** is the process of providing a constant movement of air by inspiration (inhalation) and expiration (exhalation).

   • Movement of the thorax, intercostal muscles and diaphragm determines the volume of air moved during each breath.

   • Normally, breathing is a relatively unconscious and effortless activity. Increased airway resistance and increased cellular oxygen requirements may markedly increase the ventilatory workload.

   • The primary drive for respiratory activity is a change in serum carbon dioxide levels. A decreased oxygen level is the secondary stimulus.

2. **Changes in the intrathoracic pressures** when the diaphragm and rib cage move determine airflow. The pleura permit smooth, lubricated movement of lung tissue against the thorax during respiratory activity. Normally, there is no air between the pleural layers.

   • Inspiratory activity governs the oxygen supply to the alveoli. And, exhalation governs the removal of carbon dioxide.

   • When respiratory disease obstructs airflow, intercostal and sternal retractions may occur during inhalation.

Gas Exchange Cycle Review

The cycle of exchange of oxygen and carbon dioxide begins in the alveolar sacs: (1) inspiratory phase of oxygen supply and delivery into circulation, (2) tissue/cellular consumption and metabolism, and (3) expiratory phase or the return/removal of metabolic waste products.

1. At the alveolar level, oxygen moves into the pulmonary capillaries and attaches to the hemoglobin molecule on red blood cells. Oxygenated red blood cells travel through the pulmonary veins to the left side of the heart and then into the general circulation.

   • Adequate oxygen delivery requires a sufficient number of erythrocytes and available hemoglobin molecules. Efficient pumping capacity of the myocardium, sufficient intravascular volume, and appropriate vascular resistance are essential for systemic perfusion.

2. At the peripheral tissue level, oxygen ions leave the capillaries in sufficient quantities for aerobic cellular metabolism. An insufficient oxygen supply at the cellular level triggers the conversion of metabolism to a less effective anaerobic mechanism.

   • SaO_2, paO_2, and oximetry (a method of measuring SaO_2) assessment provide data on oxygen delivery.

   • SvO_2, $paCO_2$ and capnometry (a measure of CO_2) assessment provide data on oxygen utilization/consumption.

3. **Age variation:**

   • paO_2 values among the elderly normally decrease by an estimated rate of 10 mmHg per decade during the 60-90 year age span. The oxygen saturation levels remain within the normal range in spite of this decrease.

Arterial Blood Gas (ABG) Analysis

Data provided by one or a series of ABG values increase the understanding of appropriate nursing interventions and medical management of individuals with acute respiratory conditions. This unit addresses the changes in the acid-base balance related to respiratory dysfunction and metabolic compensation. The following three steps provide pertinent data from a given ABG.

Step 1: Look at the pH to determine the general acid-base state.

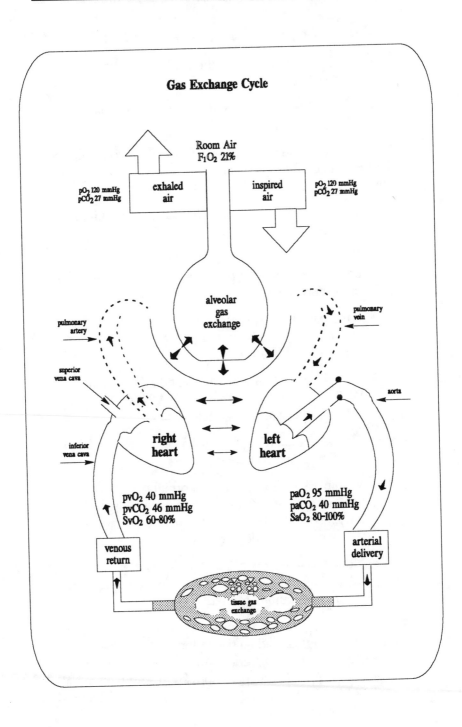

Gas Exchange Cycle

- Normal parameters (WNL) for pH: 7.35-7.45

- If the pH is below 7.35, the acid-base imbalance is acidosis.

- If the pH is above 7.45, the acid-base imbalance is alkalosis.

Step 2: Look at the $paCO_2$ and HCO_3 values to determine the type of acid-base imbalance due to respiratory pathophysiology.

- Normal parameters (WNL) for $paCO_2$ are: 35-45 mmHg.

- If the $paCO_2$ is above 45 mmHg and the pH is below 7.35, then the primary acid-base imbalance is respiratory acidosis.

- If the paCO2 is below 35 mmHg and the pH is above 7.45, then the primary acid-base imbalance is respiratory alkalosis.

- With abnormal $paCO_2$ values and HCO_3 values WNL, the acid-base imbalance is **UNCOMPENSAT-ED** respiratory acidosis or alkalosis.

Step 3: Look at the HCO_3 to determine the degree of compensation provided by the kidneys.

- Within 24-72 hours of an abnormal $paCO_2$ value, the kidneys are able to retain or generate sufficient amounts of HCO_3 ions to compensate or balance the respiratory acidosis or alkalosis.

- Normal parameters (WNL) for HCO_3 are: 22-26 mEq/L (although findings may vary according to the laboratory equipment used).

- When respiratory acidosis is present ($paCO_2$ above 45 mmHg), a gradual rise in the HCO_3 value above the normal parameter (26 mEq/L) reflects metabolic compensation. The pH also rises toward the normal (7.35). This acid-base imbalance is called **COMPEN-SATING** respiratory acidosis.

— A similar but reverse pattern of compensation occurs with a primary respiratory alkalotic state.

• When the metabolic compensation balances the respiratory imbalance, the pH will be WNL. A balance between a primary respiratory imbalance and metabolic compensation is called **COMPENSATED** respiratory acidosis or alkalosis.

• When respiratory acidosis and metabolic acidosis are present at the same time, a combined acidotic state is present. This serious imbalance is associated with a rapidly falling pH. If uncorrected, respiratory and cardiac arrest are imminent and the mortality rate is high.

Section 2: PULMONARY PATHOPHYSIOLOGY

High acuity respiratory problems develop from impaired gas exchange. To effectively manage these clinical situations and restore optimal respiratory function, an understanding of the effects and interrelationship of oxygenation, hypoxemia and hypercapnia is essential.

Hemoglobin/Oxygen Relationship

1. Hemoglobin molecules carry the majority of oxygen ions through the circulatory system. Therefore, increases or decreases in hemoglobin (Hgb) concentration affect the oxygen content in the blood (paO_2).

2. When there is less hemoglobin in circulation, the capability of transporting oxygen diminishes and the paO_2 is below normal. If the quantities of RBC and hemoglobin are low and if all available Hgb molecules are carrying oxygen ions, the saturation (SaO_2) may be WNL.

• Normal Hemoglobin (Hgb) values:
Male: 14-18g/dL;
Female: 12-16 g/dL;
Children: 13.5-18.0 g/dL

• Normal Hematocrit (Hct) values:
Male: 40-54%;

Female: 37-47%;
Children: 40-50%

- Normal RBC values:
  Male: 45-60 million/uL;
  Female: 40-55 million/uL;
  Children: 25-35 million/Kg of body weight

3. As the paO_2 decreases, an initial compensatory mechanism to low oxygen content in circulation is an increase in the heart rate and cardiac output. If cardiovascular disease is present, this mechanism may be ineffective.

4. Assessment of oxygenation requires knowledge of current values, trends, age variations for ABG's, mixed venous saturation parameters and capnometry. Assessment also includes determination of congruency between clinical manifestations and laboratory data.

Oxyhemoglobin Curve

1. A predictable pattern or curve depicts the rate of association (attachment/binding) and dissociation (release) of oxygen ions from hemoglobin molecules.

2. Oxyhemoglobin association, which occurs in the lungs, refers to the binding of oxygen ions with hemoglobin molecules. Oxyhemoglobin dissociation is the reverse process. At the cellular level, hemoglobin molecules release, or free oxygen ions.

- Several factors (acidosis, increased pCO_2) cause the curve to move to the right. When this shift occurs, there is increased release of oxygen ions at the cellular level. The pulse oximetry may reveal a low peripheral oxygen saturation value.

  — With a shift to the right, higher paO_2 values are needed to maintain aerobic metabolism (SaO_2 of 80% or better).

- Several factors (alkalosis, hyperventilation, decreased pCO_2) cause the curve to move to the left. When this shift occurs, there is increased binding of oxygen to the hemoglobin molecules in the lungs. There is an associated impaired release of oxygen at the tissue level for cellular metabolism. The pulse oximetry may reveal a relatively high peripheral oxygen saturation value.

  — A shift to the left maintains aerobic metabolism (SaO_2 at or above 80%) in spite of low paO_2 values.

Respiratory Failure

1. A sequence of pathophysiological events leads to respiratory failure. It begins with a respiratory condition that interferes with the ventilation-perfusion relationship. Tissue hypoxemia develops when decreasing amounts of oxygen are available in the circulatory system.

2. Recognition of the early stages of the respiratory failure cycle and the prompt initiation of interventions can slow the progression. Monitoring the trends in oxygenation status is essential for early recognition.

   - Inspiratory problems may lead to insufficient oxygen supply to the alveoli. If insufficient quantities of hemoglobin, RBC's or cardiac output are also present, the cells may receive inadequate quantities of oxygen leading to tissue hypoxemia. Oxygen therapy usually corrects this situation. If FiO_2 of 40% or higher is needed to restore or maintain paO_2 and SaO_2 WNL, mechanical ventilation may be indicated.

   - Expiratory problems may lead to an accumulation of carbon dioxide within the circulatory system. Without improved or effective exhalation, mechanical ventilation may be indicated.

3. One compensatory mechanism for respiratory dysfunction is an increase in the rate and depth of respiratory activity. An increase in the work of breathing also increases the metabolic rate. A cycle begins with increased oxygen consumption and carbon dioxide production.

- If not interrupted, the cycle of hypoxemia and hypercapnia worsens. As the work of breathing increases, the respiratory muscles become fatigued and hypoventilation develops.

4. As the compensatory response diminishes, respiratory failure progresses. Multisystem organ failure (MSOF) develops as hypoxemia becomes more severe. Subsequently impaired cellular metabolism occurs.

5. Age Variations

- With advanced aging, lung tissue and accessory structures lose some ability to expand and contract during the breathing cycle. Therefore, there is an estimated 45% decrease in vital capacity and 55-60% decrease in maximum breathing capacity.

- Infants and children are more likely to experience a respiratory arrest prior to a cardiac arrest. Clinical manifestations of pending respiratory arrest are subtle: flaccid skeletal muscular weakness; weak cry; poor sucking response; retractions; grunting; bradycardia for age; nasal flaring.

Lactic Acidosis

1. This is a serious complication of respiratory failure. Prolonged hypoxemia and impaired gas exchange may lead to serious cellular metabolic imbalance. Cellular metabolism converts from an aerobic to an anaerobic state.

2. Lactic acid is one of the waste products of anaerobic metabolism. Elevated serum lactic acid levels lead to increased capillary permeability. Fluid shifts between

Cycle of Respiratory Failure

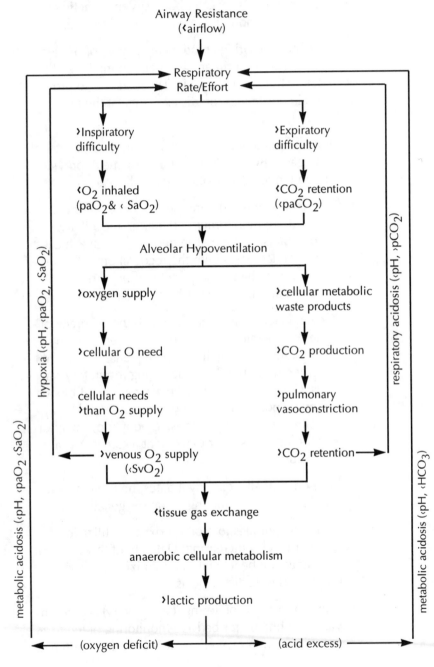

vascular and interstitial spaces further impair cellular metabolism which affects all body systems. Lactic acidosis has a high mortality rate if it is not reversed.

3. Until recently, ensuring an adequate supply of oxygen to the cells was the primary approach to minimize the development of lactic acidosis. The goal was to provide optimal circumstances for gas exchange at the tissue level.

   • Monitoring arterial oxygen saturation (SaO_2), arterial blood gas (ABG) analysis or pulse oximetry provides data on the adequacy of oxygen delivery.

   • Pulse oximetry is a noninvasive technique for continuous bedside monitoring of the arterial capillary hemoglobin saturation. The need for invasive measurements decreases with the recognition of the subtle or sudden changes in peripheral oxygen saturation and initiation of corrective interventions.

     — Several factors may interfere with the accuracy of the data obtained. For example, a person with CO_2 retention may have an adequate peripheral oxygen saturation but a declining respiratory status. Conditions which decrease peripheral blood flow (hypothermia, vasoconstriction, shock) may limit data accuracy. Excessive body movement or inappropriate sensor placement also can reveal inaccurate readings.

     — Presence of alkalosis invalidates the usefulness of oximetry in determining tissue oxygenation.

4. The use of techniques to monitor oxygen utilization at the cellular level is increasing. Data about this phase of gas exchange are beneficial in minimizing the serious consequences of lactic acidosis.

   • End Tidal CO_2 Monitoring (capnometry) is a noninvasive technique for bedside monitoring of the CO_2 concentration in expired air. It is an indirect estimate

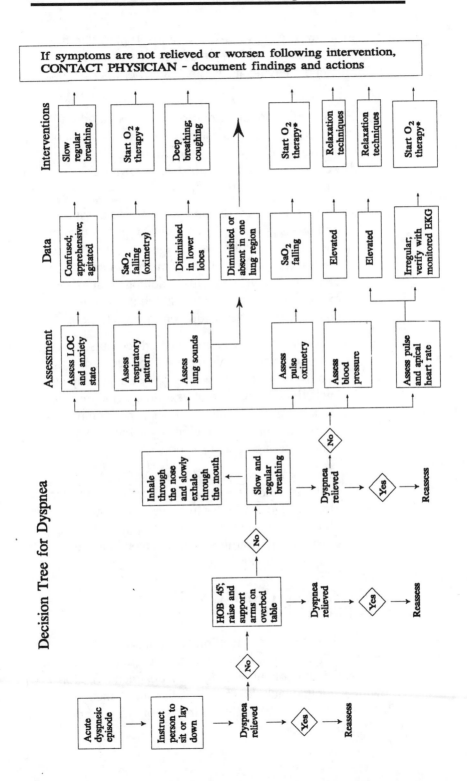

Decision Tree for Dyspnea

If symptoms are not relieved or worsen following intervention, CONTACT PHYSICIAN - document findings and actions

Interventions

Slow regular breathing

Start O₂ therapy*

Deep breathing; coughing

Start O₂ therapy*

Relaxation techniques

Relaxation techniques

Start O₂ therapy*

Data

Confused; apprehensive; agitated

SaO₂ falling (oximetry)

Diminished in lower lobes

Diminished or absent in one lung region

SaO₂ falling

Elevated

Elevated

Irregular; verify with monitored EKG

Assessment

Assess LOC and anxiety state

Assess respiratory pattern

Assess lung sounds

Assess pulse oximetry

Assess blood pressure

Assess pulse and apical heart rate

Acute dyspneic episode → Instruct person to sit or lay down → Dyspnea relieved → Yes → Reassess

No

HOB 45; raise and support arms on overbed table → Dyspnea relieved → Yes → Reassess

No

Slow and regular breathing → Dyspnea relieved → Yes → Reassess

Inhale through the nose and slowly exhale through the mouth

No

of serum $paCO_2$ values. The sensor is placed in the artificial airway or T-piece adaptor. The values obtained are typically 1-4 mmHg lower than serum (ABG) values.

- Continuous monitoring of mixed venous blood saturation (SvO_2) provides data on the oxygen saturation of the hemoglobin returning to the heart. Obtaining this data is an invasive procedure involving the insertion of an intravascular catheter.

  — Comparison of arterial and venous oxygen saturation levels permits estimation of oxygen utilization and cellular metabolism. Oxygen supply or delivery is monitored by pulse oximetry and arterial blood gases. SvO_2 provides additional data about oxygen use or consumption at the cellular level by determining oxygen saturation in venous blood.

  — SvO_2 monitoring allows the bedside nurse to determine accurately the effect of interventions on tissue oxygenation. Changes in tissue oxygenation and oxygen utilization provide the criteria for grouping interventions and planning rest periods. Prompt evaluation of the therapeutic effects of interventions is possible.

  — The normal range of SvO_2 is 60-80%. A significant deviation is a finding of more than 10% for longer than 5 minutes from an individual baseline. Factors affecting oxygen supply and tissue demand are examined and interventions are adjusted appropriately.

Section 3: RESTORATION OF GAS EXCHANGE

The ability to recognize the clinical manifestations which reflect respiratory dysfunction and altered gas exchange is an essential component of a nursing assessment. The following guideline includes representative and typical clinical manifestations. While this listing is not inclusive or exhaustive, the determination of the presence or absence of these manifestations provides a sound baseline. Obtained data are valuable in identifying nursing care diagnoses and evaluating the effectiveness of nursing interventions and medical therapies.

Guidelines of Pulmonary Assessment

1. General Appearance:

- Headache

- Lightheadedness

- Diaphoresis

- Restlessness

- Weakness

- Lethargy

- Excited/agitation

2. Respiratory Effort:

- Respiratory rate and/or depth of breaths altered

- Tachypnea (fast rate)

- Bradypnea (slow rate)

- Hyperventilation (increased depth)

- Periodic apnea

- Use of accessory muscles; intercostal and/or sternal retractions.

3. Shortness of Breath (dyspnea):

- At rest or with activity; associated changes in pulse or blood pressure.

- Position used for easier breathing (upright or supine).

- Number of pillows used when sleeping.

- Self-reporting of dyspnea severity using a 1 to 10

scale (1 = no breathing difficulty to 10 = the worst dyspneic episode experienced).

4. **Cough & Sputum Production:** amount and description.

5. **Chest Pain:** associated with any of the previous symptoms.

6. **Skin Color:** pallor; peripheral or circumoral cyanosis; temperature of extremities.

7. **Auscultated Lung Sounds:** Using the diaphragm of a stethoscope, compare right/left and anterior/posterior sounds during inspiration and expiration. The presence of adventious sounds during one phase of breathing (i.e., inspiration) that progress into the other phase (i.e., expiration) may be an early indicator of impending respiratory failure.

- If possible, have the person lie flat on his/her back for anterior auscultation. If possible, have the person sit upright so that you can auscultate both sides of the thorax at the same time for comparison of sounds in the same lung fields. If an upright position is not possible, turn the person first to one side to auscultate one side of the thorax. Then, turn the person to the opposite side to auscultate the other side. Recalling the exact sounds heard and making accurate comparison is often difficult.

  — When turning is contraindicated, listen to the lateral chest wall for additional data. Place the diaphragm of the stethoscope 2-3" below the axilla and just above the diaphragm to elicit lungs sounds from the outer portions of the underlying lobes.

- Normal vesicular sounds have a "breezy," soft, and smooth sound when auscultated during inspiration.

- Normal bronchial sounds have a "hollow" and loud or sometimes harsh sound normally auscultated over the trachea. When auscultated over the lung fields, consolidation may be present.

- Crackles ("rales") are abnormal (adventitious) breath sounds superimposed upon normal sounds. They are due to air moving through fluid in the small airways or the sudden opening of collapsed small airways. Fine crackles resemble the sound of rubbing hair between one's fingers. Coarse crackles resemble the sound of crumpling Saran Wrap or opening Velcro.

- Rhonchi are abnormal (adventitious) breath sounds superimposed upon normal sounds. They are due to fluid or mucus movement in larger airways and have a snoring or bubbling quality when auscultated during expiration.

- Wheezes are an abnormal (adventitious) breath sounds superimposed upon normal sounds. They are due to air movement through narrowed airways when auscultated during expiration. Wheezing heard during both inspiration and expiration is serious and respiratory failure is usually imminent.

Auscultating Lung Sounds

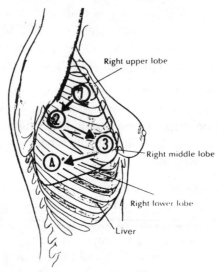

Right arm raised

Right upper lobe

Right middle lobe

Right lower lobe

Liver

Right Lateral View

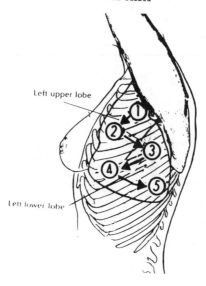

Left arm raised

Left upper lobe

Left lower lobe

Left Lateral View

MECHANICAL VENTILATION

This complex intervention provides a person in respiratory failure with mechanical support to restore and maintain adequate gas exchange through an artificial airway. An endotracheal (ET) tube inserted through the nasal or oral orifice or through a tracheostomy connects to a ventilator. To prevent displacement, twill tape, adhesive tape or commercial stabilizing devices secure the tube in place.

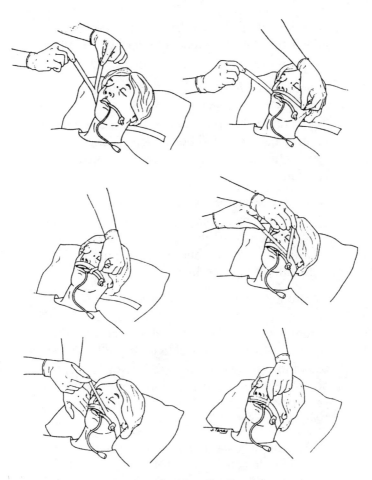

Taping the ET tube in place

Janet Beth McCann Flynn, and Nancie Purdue Bruce, Introduction to Critical Care Skills, Mosby-Year Book, 1993. Reprinted with permission.

Commonly used ventilators are either pressure-cycled (usually for small children or advanced elders) or volume-cycled (usually for adults). Professional nurses, physicians and respiratory therapists coordinate effective mechanical ventilation.

1. Common Modes of Delivery of Mechanical Ventilation:

- For volume-cycled ventilation, the following formula provides an estimation of the tidal volume (TV): 8-10 ml/kg of body weight. Using this estimation, one can determine if the TV delivered by the ventilator is adequate, or is hyperventilating or hypoventilating the person.

- Synchronized intermittent mandatory ventilation (SIMV) is a commonly prescribed mode for sustaining an optimal respiratory rate. A pre-determined respiratory rate delivered by the ventilator is synchronized with an individual's initiated inspiratory effort.

  — The individual is also able to initiate additional independent, spontaneous breaths. The actual or total respiratory rate includes the breaths delivered with the ventilator and the additional spontaneous breaths completed by the individual.

- Controlled mode ventilation (CM) provides a prescribed number of breaths per minute at a prescribed volume without stimulus from the patient. When spontaneous respiratory activity is present, effective use of this mode often requires the concurrent administration of pancuronium bromide (Pavulon) or vecuronium bromide (Norcuron), midazolam HCl (Versed), or propofol (Diprivan).

  — A neuromuscular blocking agent blocks all skeletal muscle activity including blinking of the eye, swallowing and movement of extremities. It does not block hearing, tactile, and pain sensations. Therefore, concurrent administration of sedation is required to minimize the adverse effects of these physiological and psychological stresses. As hearing remains unaffected, all physical contact and interactions should be explained prior to beginning an activity. Avoid startling the person!

- Data from paO_2 and SaO_2 serum values and peripheral oximetry offer a guideline for providing humidified oxygen with an FiO_2 between 21% (room air) to 100%. The goal is to maintain circulating oxygen WNL with the lowest FiO_2 level.

  — Use of FiO_2 > .60 for longer than 48 hours may damage the endothelial lining of the lung and decrease surfactant production (oxygen toxicity).

2. Adjunct Modes for Mechanical Ventilation:

- Peak end expiratory pressure (PEEP) is a mode used to improve gas exchange by maintaining the patency of lower air ducts and alveoli following exhalation and prior to the next inhalation. This pressure decreases the effort needed to re-inflate narrowed or collapsed passages and/or alveoli.

  — Generally PEEP pressures range from 2.5 to 10 cm H_2O. With higher pressures, there is an added risk of decreased venous return, decreased cardiac output and/or spontaneous, tension pneumothorax.

  — Continuous positive airway pressure (CPAP) functions in the same manner as PEEP. This mode requires spontaneous breathing and a T-piece adaptor.

- Pressure controlled ventilation (PCV) is a mode commonly used with small children and advanced elders during pressure-cycled ventilation. Peak inspiratory pressure (PIP) is a mode commonly used with small children and advanced elders during pressure-cycled ventilation. Maintaining airway pressure for adequate gas exchange requires a balance between PIP and PEEP.

- High frequency ventilation (HFV) utilizes rapid respiratory rate (over 60/min for adults) with small tidal volumes to achieve adequate oxygenation.

- Extra corporeal membrane oxygenation (ECMO) provides temporary cardiac/pulmonary support by using external cardiopulmonary bypass with a membrane oxygenator.

3. Complications Related to Mechanical Ventilation:

- Tension pneumothorax may develop with high volume-cycled ventilation or diseased/damaged lung tissue. In addition to the usual indicators of a pneumothorax, sudden and sustained elevated peak inspiratory pressures (PIP) occur.

- Gastric ulceration with hemorrhage may develop as a result of stress or inadequate enteral feeding. There is a risk of aspiration of gastric contents or tube feeding. Swallowed air may lead to gastric dilation and may compromise respiratory efficiency.

- High intrathoracic pressures, volume-cycled ventilation and PEEP decrease venous return to the heart. Hemodynamic monitoring detects changes and trends in decreasing cardiac output, hypotension and other perfusion deficits. Refer to Unit 4 for additional information on hemodynamic monitoring.

- Increased intracranial pressure may develop subsequent to altered systemic hemodynamics, decreased venous return and decreased cerebral perfusion.

- Nosocomial respiratory infections may occur.

4. Extubation and Weaning Guidelines:

- Assessment of eligibility for weaning for an adult is considered within 7-10 days after initiating mechanical ventilation. Secondary pressure on the tracheal wall occurs with the use of a cuffed nasal or oral intubation tube. Continuous, prolonged pressure of an inflated cuff may lead to tracheal wall ulceration and the possibility of tracheal-esophageal fistula formation.

— If weaning cannot be achieved within a 7-10 day interval, a tracheostomy is performed to deliver mechanical ventilation.

• Weaning from mechanical ventilation begins with a plan for decreasing one of the following ventilator settings at scheduled small increments: FiO_2, SIMV rate or PEEP. Comparisons between current and pre-adjustment physical condition, venous saturation and ABG's determine the rate of weaning to meet and maintain established criteria.

• For trial nonmechanical ventilation, a T-piece adaptor is used prior to removing the ET tube. Strength and endurance of independent respiratory activity are progressively achieved. Return to mechanical support is easily accomplished without the need for re-intubation.

— The T-piece adaptor provides humidified oxygen and CPAP may be added to prevent alveolar collapse.

— Progressive weaning usually begins with an hourly schedule of spontaneous, independent breathing for 2-5 minutes and 55-58 minutes with SIMV ventilator breathing. The length of ventilator breathing is gradually decreased reversing the ratio. Independent breathing while awake is usually achieved before independent breathing while sleeping.

5. Criteria for Extubation and/or Weaning:

• Spontaneous respiratory activity with TV appropriate for body weight (5-10 ml/Kg) and negative respiratory force -20 or greater

- Adequate nutritional status (serum albumin > 2.5 g/dL)

- PEEP less than 5 cm H_2O

- FiO_2 less than 35%

- ABG values WNL or close to patient's baseline ABGs

6. Troubleshooting Ventilator Problems:

- The most important aspect of care for an individual receiving mechanical ventilation is the effect that this treatment has on the individual patient. Do not depend only on the ventilator settings or alarm sounds, always assess the person to determine his/her physiological response.

- High pressure alarms indicating increased airway resistance may sound when: (1) endotracheal suctioning is needed, (2) kinks, secretions, or water occurs in the tubing between the ventilator and the person, (3) person coughs against a ventilator delivered breath, or (4) person bites the oral ET tube.

- Low pressure alarm may sound with: (1) an inadequate connection between the ET tube and the ventilator tubing, (2) a leaking endotracheal/airway cuff, or (3) a displaced ET tube above the vocal cords.

7. Communication Difficulty:

- An individual receiving mechanical ventilation may also be conscious, oriented and able to hear and understand. Being unable to communicate one's needs and concerns is very stressful and frustrating. Concrete statements to orient the individual to his/her surroundings, current time and care activities are essential. Care interventions should NOT be initiated without an explanation

- Inquiries directed to the person should be phrased for "yes" or "no" responses or communicated for an eyeblinking or finger-raising responses. For example, a "yes" response may be one eyeblink or one raised finger and a "no" response may be two eyeblinks or two raised fingers. All health care personnel should use the same response indicator when interacting with the person.

- A slateboard or notepad is helpful for more detailed communication. Picture boards conveying commonly used activities, such as the word "pain" or a picture of a bedpan are helpful for a person whose handwriting is difficult to read.

8. Age Variations:

- Adult artificial airways must have a cuff that is inflated to establish a closed system for effective mechanical ventilation.

- Neonate and small pediatric ET tubes do not require cuffs because the cricoid cartilage of an infant or child is pliable and provides a sufficient seal around an inserted tube.

- Physiological pulmonary changes associated with aging may delay the weaning from mechanical ventilation for elderly persons. Elders are also prone to atelectasis and pneumonia.

  — NOTE: Fever is often undetected among the elderly as their body temperature is typically lower than younger persons.

Additional Interventions to Improve Pulmonary Function

1. Thoracentesis:

- When the inner or visceral pleura are lacerated or punctured, air escapes into the pleural space with each inhalation. The accumulating trapped air compresses and collapses the underlying lung tissue (tension pneumothorax). The trapped air rises toward the top of the pleural space of the thorax.

— A large gauge needle is typically inserted in the
second midclavicular intercostal space and into
the underlying pleural space to relieve the accumulated air. Inserted chest tubes maintain
intrathoracic pressures.

• When fluid collects in the pleural space, it settles at the
base of the pleural space.

— For chest-tube insertion, the person is placed in
an upright sitting position, arms are raised,
crossed and placed on a raised bed table. Rest
the head on folded arms to extend the chest wall.
The site of insertion depends on the location and
volume of fluid. Typically, the site is lateral posterior between the 6th-8th ribs.

2. Chest Tube Insertion:

• Guidelines for insertion of chest tubes are similar to
needle insertion for a thoracocentesis. An anteriorly
inserted tube removes accumulated air. A posteriorly
inserted tube removes accumulated fluid from the
lower pleural space.

• One to three bottle set up or commercially available
combined single unit removes accumulated fluid.
The fluid level should rise in the tube with inspiration and fall with expiration. This fluctuation occurs
until the lung re-expansion occurs. Chest x-ray verifies re-expansion before tube removal.

— Under-water seal is a one-bottle closed system
attached to the inserted tube. Suction is administered with caution as it can accentuate the air
leak.

— Deep breathing facilitates lung expansion.
Coughing is discouraged when a pleural air leak
is present.

— Clamping chest tubes is controversial. If a pleural
air leak is present, a clamped chest tube may permit inspired air to move through the air leak into

the pleural space and may extend the pneumoth-orax.

— Heimlich flutter valve is an alternative to a water-seal drainage. A valve allows drainage while preventing reflux of air or fluid back into the pleural space.

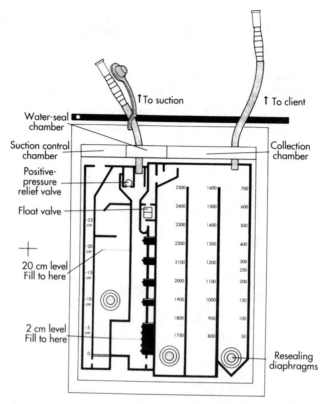

Pleur-evac disposable chest suction system. From S.M. Lewis, I.C. Collier. Medical-Surgical Nursing: Assessment and Management of Clinical Problems, 3rd ed. St. Louis: Mosby-Year Book, 1992. Reprinted with permission.

— The under-water seal is a one-bottle closed system attached to the inserted tube. Suction is administered with caution as it can accentuate the air leak.

— Deep breathing facilitates lung expansion. Coughing is discouraged when a pleural air leak is present.

— Clamping chest tubes is controversial. If pleural air leak is present, a clamped chest tube may permit inspired air to move through the air leak into the pleural space and may extend the pneumothorax.

— The Heimlich flutter valve is an alternative to a water-sealed drainage. A valve allows drainage while preventing reflux of air or fluid back into the pleural space.

- Removing a chest tube may be painful. The administration of an adequate dose of analgesia 30 minutes prior to removal is recommended. After cutting the suture which secured the tube, the person is asked to inhale deeply as the tube is promptly removed. A Telfa dressing covers the insertion site to ensure an airtight covering. Respiratory activity and oxygenation are evaluated.

3. Endotracheal Suctioning:

- Sterile technique is used for removing secretions from the air passages through an artificial airway. Guidelines for maintaining airway clearance include:

    — Wear gloves and goggles as universal precautions against contaminated blood and body fluids.

    — Oxygenate ventilated persons with FiO_2 at 100% and hyperventilation before and following suctioning. Hypoxemia may occur if the ventilatory system is disconnected during suctioning. A closed suction system is the preferred method when maintaining continuous oxygenation and PEEP are essential.

    — Duration and frequency of suctioning passes are dependent upon the quantity of secretions and changes in oxygenation status. Monitor oxygen supply and cellular need through SaO_2/pulse oximetry and SvO_2/capnometry.

    — Use sterile disposable equipment as the risk of nosocomial pneumonia is increased with artificial airways.

    — Stop suctioning if bradycardia or ectopy occur. Provide supplemental oxygen at 100% FiO_2 to restore normal sinus rhythm.

    — Periodic instillation of 2-3 ml of sterile saline into an adult ET tube prior to suctioning liquifies thick secretions for easier removal and decreases the risk of mucosal injury. Frequent instillation of sterile saline in quantities larger than 2-3 ml may dilute or "wash out" surfactant resulting in collapsed alveoli.

Section 4: EXAMPLES OF COMMON HIGH ACUITY CLINICAL CONDITIONS

Adult Respiratory Distress Syndrome (ARDS)

This condition is not a primary condition but results secondarily from altered circulatory perfusion to the lung tissue. Thus, it is commonly called "shock lung."

1. Pathophysiology:

- A variety of pathophysiological causes may injure the alveolar-capillary membrane. There is increased permeability and fluid shifts between the pulmonary capillaries and alveoli. An accumulation of protein-rich fluid develops within the alveolar walls and inside the alveoli which interferes with gas exchange. In addition, there is a reduction in surfactant activity and alveoli collapse.

- When pulmonary circulation improves, the blood passes through the pulmonary capillaries, but gas exchange is inadequate. Right-to-left pulmonary shunting occurs.

  — Hypoxia due to right-to-left shunting does not improve with oxygen administration. Additional FiO_2 administration is unable to cross the alveolar-capillary membrane

- There is a marked increase in ventilatory effort to inflate collapsed alveoli and permit gas exchange across the fluid filled alveoli. While chest movement and visible breathing occurs, ineffective alveolar gas exchange exits.

- As hypoxemia increases, anaerobic cellular metabolism occurs and lactic acid accumulates in the blood. Lactic acidosis increases capillary permeability and furthers the fluid leakage within alveolar tissue. If unresponsive to therapy, the cycle of injured alveoli, fluid filled or collapsed alveoli and impaired gas exchange result in a high mortality rate.

2. Indications:

- Decreasing paO_2 value that is unresponsive to increasing FiO_2 administration.

- Serial chest x-rays reveal diffuse infiltrate. As the condition progresses, there is an increasing white appearance to the lung fields. Fewer air spaces remain useful for gas exchange.

- As the condition worsens, effective exhalation diminishes leading to accumulated carbon dioxide in circulation (respiratory acidosis).

- Clinical assessment findings reveal the degree of impaired gas exchange (hypoxia and hypercapnia) and evolving acidosis.

3. Medical and Nursing Management:

- If respiratory failure develops, mechanical ventilation is initiated. Positive inspiratory and expiratory pressure maintain patent lower airducts. If the person has adequate spontaneous breathing, CPAP is used. PEEP is used if mechanical ventilation is required.

- For premature infants, surfactant replacement therapy reduces the severity of the consequences of respiratory failure. Protocols are being tested for ARDS (adults).

- Intravenous fluid therapy maintains an adequate cardiac output with a minimum pulmonary artery wedge pressure (PAWP). This balance provides adequate perfusion to the lungs without producing an intracapillary pressure that would add to the fluid leakage in the alveoli.

- Nutritional support is necessary because of the high energy expenditure required to breathe during respiratory failure. The early initiation of enteral feedings or parenteral nutrition minimizes a negative nitrogen balance and maintains a serum albumin level of 2.5 g/dL.

Acute Episode of Chronic Obstructive Pulmonary Disease (COPD)

Chronic obstructive lung disease (COLD) is another term currently used for this syndrome. It is a primary cause for disability in the United States.

COPD/COLD is a constellation of three respiratory conditions: asthma, chronic bronchitis, and emphysema. These conditions interrelate and lead to progressive lung damage. A chronic state of respiratory acidosis with compensated metabolic alkalosis is the typical, balanced acid-base state for an individual with COPD/COLD. However, the development of a relatively minor secondary condition often upsets the balance leading to an acute episode of respiratory failure.

1. Pathophysiology:

- Generally accepted criteria for respiratory failure are: paO_2 <50 mmHg, $paCO_2$ >50 mmHg and SaO_2 <85%.

  — NOTE: The respiratory drive for individuals with COPD is no longer an elevated $paCO_2$ value but a low paO_2 value (an hypoxic respiratory drive). Administering oxygen greater than 2-4 L/min may block this individual's stimulus for spontaneous and adequate respirations resulting in apnea.

- While individuals with COPD/COLD usually have $paCO_2$ values of 50 mmHg, their paO_2 and SaO_2 are within a low normal range. The renal system is able to retain and produce sufficient amounts of HCO_3 (bicarbonate) ions to balance the chronic elevated CO_2 (acidotic) ions; the result is compensated respiratory acidosis.

— If the kidneys are unable to produce sufficient HCO_3 ions in circulation, the elevated $paCO_2$ values will produce an uncompensated respiratory acidotic state. This imbalance may occur with a secondary renal/urinary condition, i.e., benign prostatic hypertrophy (BPH) or urinary tract infection (UTI).

• While individuals with COPD/COLD usually have low but adequate paO_2 and SaO_2 levels, retained pulmonary secretions may become infected and quickly alter gas exchange. Hypoxemia (paO_2 < 50 mmHg) and inadequate serum oxygen saturation (SaO_2 < 85%) will lead to anaerobic cellular metabolism. Subsequent lactic acidosis, with an underlying respiratory acidosis, results in a rapidly falling serum pH and a profound combined acidotic state.

• Air filled bubbles may develop with advanced emphysema. When these bubbles occur on the surface of the lung, they are called blebs. Bullae are air-filled bubbles that occur within lung tissue. Sudden changes in intralung pressure (severe coughing) can rupture blebs or bullae causing a spontaneous, tension pneumothorax.

• Pulmonary capillary vasoconstriction and pulmonary hypertension accompany a chronic state of respiratory acidosis. Subsequently, there is a back-up or congestion in the right ventricle of the heart. This condition is called right-sided congestive heart failure secondary to a pulmonary condition or cor pulmonale.

— The clinical symptoms of cor pulmonale are treated with cardiotonic glycosides (digitalis), diuretics, potassium replacements and sodium restriction. (For additional discussion on congestive heart failure (CHF) refer to Unit 4: Care of Individuals with High Acuity Cardiac Conditions.)

2. Medical and Nursing Management:

- Mechanical ventilation not only corrects abnormal gas exchange but also decreases the effort to breathe. This situation presents a secondary problem for persons with COPD/COLD as their spontaneous respiratory activity typically requires increased effort and energy expenditure. Weaning from mechanical ventilation following an acute episode of respiratory failure often becomes a long, slow process.

- Knowing the person's pre-episode gas exchange state is helpful to individualize the parameters for mechanical ventilation. Achieving textbook blood gas values is usually not realistic.

- Treatment and correction of the secondary condition which precipitated respiratory failure are essential. Patient education, discharge planning, and case management minimize the reoccurrence of precipitating factors and rehospitalization.

3. Age Variations:

- With the aging process, there is an increased incidence of osteoporosis which may lead to changes in vertebral alignment (kyphosis) or compression fractures. These changes may decrease an elder's vital capacity and effectual cough response.

- Chronic obstructive syndrome among infants and children is usually secondary to idiopathic respiratory disease in premature infants (IRDS), bronchopulmonary dysplasia (BPD) or cystic fibrosis (CF).

Chest Trauma

Flail chest is a severe complication of blunt chest trauma when three or more adjacent ribs are fractured. The affected section of the chest moves independently and paradoxically to intrathoracic pressure. When the affected segment of the chest wall retracts in response to inhalation and bulges to exhalation, this condition is suspected.

1. Pathophysiology:

- Secondary injury to the underlying lung tissue may occur. Penetration of rib fragments into the pleural space may result in a tension pneumothorax. Thoracentesis or the insertion of chest tubes may be required.

- Secondary bruising (contusion) of lung tissue and associated inflammatory edema of surrounding tissue may lead to ARDS.

2. Medical and Nursing Management:

- Pain control is essential as fractured ribs move with each respiration producing shallow breathing, inadequate alveolar expansion and impaired gas exchange.

- The administration of humidified oxygen therapy restores and maintains peripheral oxygen saturation levels above 85% and serum paO_2 levels above 60 mmHg.

- If gas exchange remains inadequate, mechanical ventilation is initiated. PEEP, PIP and high tidal volumes maintain optimal airway pressure and stabilize the chest wall. Usually the chest wall stabilizes within 10-14 days and weaning from mechanical ventilation is possible.

- Good pulmonary hygiene for a bedfast individual will prevent the development of secondary pulmonary and immobility complications such as pneumonia, nosocomial infections, or thrombophlebitis.

Near Drowning

The description of this clinical condition is the survival for longer than 24 hours following asphyxia related to submersion. Alcohol or drug intoxication, diving injuries, seizures, or myocardial infarctions precede many adult drownings or near drownings. The accidental submersion in backyard swimming pools, ponds, or bathtubs accompany many childhood drownings or near drownings.

1. Pathophysiology:

- The interrelationship among hypoxia, hypercapnia, hypotension, and pulmonary edema results in respiratory and metabolic acidosis. Submersion in cold water may produce hypothermia with a decrease in core body temperature to 33° C (91.4° F). Cellular metabolism decreases with low core body temperature and protects hypoxic-sensitive neural tissue from damage.

  — It is recommended to continue resuscitation efforts until the core temperature raises to at least 32° C (90° F) as the heart may resume beating when warmer. Successful resuscitations have been reported even after 30 minutes of submersion in freezing water.

- Near drowning with aspiration occurs with 85-90% of the victims. The aspirant is either the submersion fluid or gastric contents. Secondary pneumonia or chemical pneumonitis usually develops.

  — Freshwater (hypotonic) aspiration results in a loss of surfactant as the pressure of the aspirated fluid moves through the alveoli and into the pulmonary circulation. With a decrease in surfactant, affected alveoli collapse and varying degrees of right-to-left shunting occurs.

  — Saltwater (hypertonic) aspiration results in a rapid shift of fluid from the pulmonary circulation into the alveoli. Inadequate ventilation occurs in these fluid filled alveoli.

- Near drowning without aspiration occurs in only 10-15% of the victims. Profound laryngospasm occurs in response to the fluid entering the airway and respiratory activity ceases. Because this breath holding response may not terminate before the systemic oxygen supply reaches dangerous low levels, dysrhythmias, seizures or death from hypoxia can occur.

2. Medical and Nursing Management:

- As ARDS sequela occurs with near drowning situations, the management of care is similar to that implemented for respiratory failure.

- Varying degrees of cerebral hypoxia may develop. Sufficient FiO_2 administration ensures optimal paO_2 and SaO_2 values.

Status Asthmaticus

Hyperactive bronchial airways associated with asthma respond to a variety of irritants with diffuse narrowing (bronchospasm), mucosal edema, and increased tenacious mucus production. If these pathophysiological responses are not reversed nor respond to medical therapies within 24 hours, status asthmaticus develops.

1. Indications:

- The process begins with coughing, chest tightness and expiratory wheezing. As gas exchange becomes impaired, labored breathing, dyspnea, fatigue, and restlessness develop.

  — Severe bronchial constriction affects both inspiratory and expiratory phases. When wheezing is absent and marked dyspnea is present, respiratory arrest is imminent.

- Clinical findings associated with impaired gas exchange initially include: prolonged expiratory phase, expiratory wheezing, hypotension, tachypnea, and tachycardia. Findings associated with ineffective inspiration include signs of hypoxia (restlessness, diaphoresis, pallor, and circumoral cyanosis).

- The paO_2 initially is WNL and then decreases as the condition becomes more severe. Usually the $paCO_2$ decreases in the early stages due to increased respiratory rate (hyperventilation). When the $paCO_2$ is normal or elevated, respiratory failure is imminent and mechanical ventilation may be warranted.

2. Medical and Nursing Management:

- Obtaining serum theophylline levels on admission determines the possibility of toxic effects from self-treatment during the early stages of an asthmatic attack. Acceptable therapeutic range is 10-20 ug/ml.

  — Clinical signs of toxicity include: nausea, restlessness, agitation, CNS stimulation, and cardiac dysrhythmias (tachycardia with PVC or PAC). Frequent serial peak and trough theophylline levels monitor the physical response to therapies and determine the titration of IV medication dosage.

- Due to the possibility of dysrhythmias, cardiac monitoring is recommended during IV theophylline administration.

- The administration of humidified oxygen therapy by nasal cannula corrects hypoxia and compensates for the increased oxygen demands and the increased workload of breathing.

- Pharmacological therapy includes bronchodilators, corticosteroids, sedatives, and antibiotics.

  — Acute adrenal insufficiency may occur if the person was taking steroids routinely at home and does not receive this medication during hospitalization. Signs of acute adrenal crisis are falling blood pressure, serum sodium and potassium imbalances, and shock.

- Intravenous access provides the route for fluid replacement and administration of medications.

- Mechanical ventilation may be required if respiratory acidosis is unresponsive to chest physiotherapy or if respiratory failure occurs.

Pulmonary Perfusion Disorders

Obstruction of the pulmonary blood flow usually occurs suddenly when an embolus travels within the venous system to the vascular bed in the lungs and obstructs a pulmonary arteriole. The degree of perfusion deficit and impaired gas exchange depends upon the size or number of vessels occluded.

1. Pathophysiology:

- Perfusion of the lung tissue distal or beyond the point of occlusion initially becomes ischemic. If the cellular metabolism is severely impaired, the affected area becomes infarcted and lung tissue dies. Surrounding tissue becomes inflamed and edematous. The size of the vessel obstruction, secondary inflammation and degree of impaired gas exchange determine the severity of symptoms. The size of tissue involvement and response to early treatment determine the recovery/mortality rate.

  — Pulmonary embolus (PE) is the most common pulmonary perfusion deficit. This condition typically occurs when a fragment of a blood clot in the lower extremities or pelvis becomes dislodged and travels to the pulmonary circulation where it occludes a branch of the pulmonary artery.

  — The cause of a fat embolus is the release of free fatty acids or bone marrow fragments into the circulation. This complication of a long bone fracture usually occurs within 48 hours following injury.

  — Less common causes include emboli released from infective colonization in the right heart chambers, tumor fragments, and amniotic fluid.

Focused Bedside Assessment

The following is a guideline of data expected from a head-to-toe assessment of an adult experiencing an acute, severe respiratory problem. Pulmonary embolis is used as one example. No other pathophysiological problems involving other body system dysfunction unrelated to this acute respiratory condition are included.

- **General appearance:** acute physical distress; verbalizes something serious has happened. Pallor, diaphoresis with cold/clammy extremities.

- **Neurological status:** restlessness, anxiety. Usually oriented but focused on present with short attention span. Confusion and/or disorientation may develop as impaired gas exchange and inadequate cerebral perfusion develop.

- **Respiratory status:** marked increase in respiratory rate (tachypnea) with the rate greater than 20 breaths/min. Nonproductive cough. Hemoptysis if infarction is present. Oppressive chest pain that does not radiate to upper extremities and is not relieved with bedrest. Chooses high Fowler's position to facilitate breathing. Petechiae on the torso and axillae usually appear with the occurrence of fat emboli. Lung fields are clear initially with the onset of adventitious sounds as inflammation of surrounding tissue develops.

- **Cardiac status:** marked and sudden onset of increased heart rate (tachycardia) with the rate >100 beats/minute. Increased blood pressure initially and may drop to shock parameters if a large arteriole is obstructed. S_3 and S_4 gallop cardiac sounds may be heard.

- **Abdominal status:** soft with no distension. Bowel sounds diminish and are absent if signs of shock develop.

- **Urinary/Renal status:** urinary output is appropriate for intake but may decrease due to diaphoresis or with the onset of shock.

- **Extremities:** appropriate movement of extremities. Usually appear pale and cool, clammy to touch. Pedal pulses unchanged.

- When this person is turned on his/her side, the nurse would expect to find that petechiae may also appear on the back or the chest.

If additional data are observed, a more detailed assessment of the involved system is required. Additional areas of physiological dysfunction may be present and confound the present respiratory problem.

2. Medical and Nursing Management:

- Position for comfort and ease in breathing; usually bedrest with high Fowler's or orthopneic position.

- Frequent arterial blood gases determine the guidelines for the initiation and adjustment of interventions.

- The administration of humidified oxygen therapy maintains a paO_2 at $\geq$ 60 mmHg. Physical activity is monitored by peripheral oxygen saturation to ensure a $SaO_2 \geq$ 85%.

- Anticoagulation therapy is immediately initiated for persons without bleeding or coagulation disorders. Recent prothrombin time (PT), partial thromboplastin time (PTT), and platelet counts provide a baseline of the current coagulation status.

  — The purpose of anticoagulation therapy is to minimize the extension or release of the existing clot or additional fragments from the original site as well as minimizing the extension of the embolus in the pulmonary arteriole.

- IV Heparin is the most common medication prescribed. Initial dosage for IV bolus is 5,000 to 10,000 units. Continued therapy includes administration every 2-4 hours or by continuous infusion. The dosage is titrated or adjusted to maintain the PTT, at 1.5-2.5 times the normal value. (Normal activated values: 30-40 seconds although values may vary according to laboratory equipment used.)

  — Protamine sulfate is the antidote for Heparin and should be readily available during therapeutic Heparin therapy. Hemorrhage during therapy has been reported and the risk is greatest in elderly women.

- Oral anticoagulant (warfarin sodium) therapy begins within 48-72 hours after the initiation of Heparin and often administered concurrently for 6-7 days before Heparin is discontinued. This regime inhibits the vitamin K-dependent clotting factors and maintains a continuous level of anticoagulation. The PT is obtained regularly for dosage adjustments to maintain the PT at 1-1.5 times normal value. (Normal values: 10-15 seconds; although values may vary according to laboratory equipment used.)

  — Vitamin K preparations reverse the anticoagulation effects of warfarin in 24-36 hours. Fresh frozen plasma may be required if serious bleeding occurs. As warfarin crosses the placenta barrier, spontaneous abortion with hemorrhage may occur.

- Thrombolytic therapy may be used for lysis of clot formation in a major pulmonary arteriole. Treatment must be initiated within 24-72 hours of the pulmonary emboli formation. There is a risk of hemorrhagic complications with this therapy.

- Monitoring for the possible onset of secondary complications facilitates the prompt initiation of corrective interventions. Pulmonary edema may develop following the occurrence of fat embolus. Impaired perfusion (shock) and respiratory failure may develop.

Pneumonia

This acute inflammation of lung tissue may be due to an infection or aspiration of gastric contents. Most cases are community-acquired and seldom require hospitalization unless there is an associated medical condition. Hospital-associated (nosocomial) cases usually develop while being hospitalized for the treatment of another medical condition. Aspiration of gastric secretions and inadequate ventilation following general surgery are also common causes.

Immunosuppression and neutropenia are predisposing factors in the development of pneumonia.

1. Indications:

- Typical clinical manifestations include: fever, cough, sputum, chest pain, dyspnea and general sense of not feeling well (malaise).

    — Elderly individuals may exhibit more subtle symptoms. Fever (>100° F) is rarely present unless the pneumonia process is severe. Impaired gas exchange will cause confusion and lethargy as presenting symptoms.

    — Early in the course of this pulmonary infection, young children develop high fever (>102° F), loud cough, and inability to sleep.

    — Typical bacteria, viruses, fungi and protozoa infect severely immunocompromised individuals. Pneumocystosis carinii pneumonia may occur in individuals with AIDS or those receiving long-term immunosuppression therapy (organ transplantation).

- A change in amount and/or character of sputum production in an intubated, ventilated individual is often the early indicator of pneumonia.

2. Medical and Nursing Management:

- Sputum specimens should be obtained prior to the initiation of antibiotic therapy. The results from culture and sensitivity testing determine the adjustments in the type and dosage of antibiotic regime.

- A hospital-acquired infection often adds at least 7-10 days to one's hospital stay. In these days of cost containment and conservation of resources, preventive interventions are cost saving to the person as well as the hospital.

- Methicillin-resistant staphylococcus aureus (MRSA) is a serious and virulent infection that most antibiotics cannot eliminate. It is important to prevent the occurrence and transmission of this infection as it is difficult to eradicate once it develops in a clinical setting. Strict handwashing for all personnel entering the person's room and aseptic technique when suctioning are needed. To minimize cross-infection and transmission, many institutional infection control guidelines recommend strict isolation of MRSA patients. Recommendations also include that health care personnel caring for a person with MRSA do not care for other persons

- Drug resistent infections are increasing and becoming life threatening. Methicillin resistant staphylococcus aureaus (MRSA) is seen as an active disease process in acute care, home health, and nursing home settings especially among ventilatory dependent persons. Vancomycin is the antibiotic of choice for drug resistant infections. However, organisms are becoming resistant to this drug and other serious infections result. VRE refers to vancomycin resistant enterococci infections and no antibiotic is currently effective in treating this life-threatening infection.

- The presence of drug resistant organisms have been found in individuals who do not have clinical symptoms. Colonization refers to the process by which these organisms are present in a symptom free individual but can be passed on to a susceptible individual. Colonization presents a significant health problem in the control of drug resistant infections.

- Blood cultures may be indicated for persistent elevated temperatures. They should be obtained prior to the initiation of antibiotic therapy.

- Mechanical ventilation may be indicated if respiratory failure develops.

- Pneumonia may lead to septicemia and septic shock. Refer to Unit 4: Nursing Care of Individuals with High Acuity Circulatory Conditions for additional information.

Acquired Immune Deficiency Syndrome (AIDS)

Acquired Immune Deficiency Syndrome (AIDS) is a life-threatening illness caused by the human immunodeficiency virus (HIV). A person who is positive to HIV but does not exhibit the symptoms of AIDS has "HIV disease." With HIV disease, the virus is circulating in the body but is unable to penetrate the body cells. The individual's immune system is able to combat the virus and keep the viral levels low. During this state, the person is a lifelong carrier and is able to transmit the virus to others. In addition, a person can be infected with the virus and be negative in blood testing, especially during the early stages of the infection. Although the virus has been found in the blood as early as one week after exposure, the majority of cases seroconvert between 6-18 weeks (95% within 3 months; 99% within 6 months).

While the virus has been isolated from blood, semen, vaginal secretions, saliva, tears, breast milk, cerebrospinal fluid, amniotic fluid, and urine, the epidemiological evidence has implicated only blood, semen, vaginal secretions, spinal fluid, and breast milk in transmission. However, the CDC recommends that barrier precautions be used for all body fluids except sweat. The human behaviors believed to be directly involved with the transmission of HIV are the following:

- Sexual intercourse with an infected person

- Sharing needles with an infected person

- An infected woman to her baby during pregnancy

- Receiving blood transfusions of infected blood (a low risk since blood screening began in 1985)

Until recently, the assessment of the helper T-cell was the primary measurement of the disease process. The CD4+T lymphocyte count continues to be predictor of the rate of disease progression and the predictor of the risk for opportunistic infections. The assessment of viral load or the quantity of circulating virus is now the best indicator of the response to drug therapy and the severity of the disease. By achieving a sustained suppression of the plasma viral load, the HIV+ person is able to resist infections and carry out all daily activities. The period of clinical latency is prolonged.

As the CD4 drops and the viral loads increase, the body's ability to fight off infection increases. When the CD4 falls below 200/mm. the possibility that an infection will be fatal increases. As the immunosuppression progresses, opportunistic infections occur which include:

- Fungal: candidiasis of bronchi, trachea, lungs or esophagus; disseminated or extrapulmonary histoplasmosis

- Viral: Cytomegalovirus (CMV) disease other than liver, spleen or nodes; CMV retinitis (with progressive loss of vision); herpes simplex with chronic ulcer(s) or bronchitis, pneumonitis or esophagitis; progressive multifocal leukoencephalopathy (PML), extrapulmonary cryptococcosis

- Protozoal: disseminated or extrapulmonary coccidiomycosis; toxoplasmosis of the brain; Pneumoncystis carinii pneumonia (PCP); chronic intestinal isosporiasis; chronic intestinal cryposporidiosis

- Bacterial: Mycobacterium tuberculosis (any site); any disseminated or extrapulmonary Mycobacterium including M. Avium complex or M. Kansasii; recurrent Salmonella septicemia

In addition to the development of opportunistic infections, opportunistic cancers may also develop. These malignant conditions include: invasive cervical carcinoma, Karposi's sarcoma (KS), Burkitt's lymphoma, immunoblastic lymphoma, or primary lymphoma of the brain. These conditions are debilitating and typically do not respond favorably to standard oncology therapies. A wasting syndrome develops in which 10% or more of an individual's ideal body mass is lost.

The treatment of HIV/AIDS is directed toward prolonging the clinical latency period and thereby delaying the onset of opportunistic infections and cancer. Current multiple drug regimes are producing sustained suppression of plasma viral loads. The recommended drug regime includes one highly active protease inhibitor and two nucleoside reverse transcriptase inhibitors (NRTI). While these drug regimes are very expensive (often $1000+/month), the person is able to maintain meaningful life. Because each drug is potent with specific intake requirements and has a high risk for adverse effects, regular monitoring of plasma response is essential. With the development of adverse effects or a rise in viral counts, the combination of drugs will vary.

Currently available protease inhibitors are:

- Crixivan (indinavir)

- Norvir (ritonavir)

- Invirase (saquinavir)

- Viracept (nelfinvir)

Currently available nucleoside reverse transcriptase inhibitors are:

- Retrovir (Zidovudine, AZT, ZDV)

- Videx (didanosine, ddl)

- HIVID (zalcitabine, ddC)

- Zerit (stavudine, d4T)

- Epivir (lamivudine, 3TC)

- Viramune (nevirapine)

- Rescriptor (delavirdine)

A common protocol for medical management includes:

1. Establishing a baseline with a CD4 (to assess the rate of disease progression), HIV-1 by PCR (to assess the viral load), a chem-enzyme panel, and a CBC. A multi-drug regime which includes one protease inhibitor and two nucleoside reverse transcriptase inhibitors is initiated. Often the CD4 and HIV-1 by PCR are repeated one week later.

2. At 4 weeks after initiating drug therapy, the CD4 and HIV-1 by PCR are repeated. There should be a 10 fold decrease in the viral load with 4 weeks of therapy.

3. Every 3 months, a CD4, HIV-1 by PCR, chem-enzyme panel and CBC are drawn. The HIV-RNA should not be detectable in the blood by 6 months of therapy. If the virus is still detectable, the USPHS Guidelines "Considerations or Changing a Failing Regime" are followed.

For more information, contact the AIDS Hotline:

1-800-342-AIDS (2437)

1-800-334-7432 (Spanish)

Unit 3

Care of Individuals with High Acuity Cardiac Conditions

This unit addresses a variety of high acuity cardiovascular conditions associated with varying degrees of impaired cardiac function and circulation. Persons with these conditions have traditionally been treated in critical care units. However, as the trends in health care delivery shift to ambulatory, extended, and home health settings, the principles of high acuity nursing care and related nursing interventions will extend beyond the walls of the traditional acute care hospital.

A knowledge of general medical-surgical nursing is basic to an understanding of the information presented in this unit. Prerequisite understanding includes normal anatomical considerations, cardiac impulse transmission, and assessment of uncomplicated cardiac status. The extension, elaboration, and refinement of these concepts provide the foundation for the nursing care of high acuity cardiac conditions.

Section 1: REVIEW AND OVERVIEW

The human heart is an amazing structure. It is estimated that an adult heart beats 72 times per minute or 100,000 times each day to circulate 1800 gallons of blood. This circulatory process is crucial for optimal cellular metabolism.

Cardiopulmonary function is the coordination between the lungs as an adequate oxygen supplier and the heart as an effective pump. Perfusion, on the other hand, is the actual distribution of oxygenated blood throughout the systemic vascular system.

Anatomical Review:

The cardiovascular system consists of an efficient pump (heart), an elaborate interconnecting system of tubing (blood vessels), and efficient carriers of the nutrients for cellular metabolism (blood components).

1. **The heart** is a master pump which is divided into four chambers which are separated by valves.

   • Functions of the heart divide in two categories according to each side of the heart. The right side of the heart receives blood from the venous system and circulates it to the lungs. The left side of the heart receives oxygenated blood from the lungs and pumps it into the systemic circulation.

2. **The vascular system** includes arteries, veins, and capillaries.

   • Arteries carry oxygenated blood from the heart to the peripheral tissue and veins carry the waste products of cellular metabolism from the tissue back to the heart and lungs. There are two exceptions: the pulmonary vein carries oxygenated blood from the lungs to the left atrium of the heart and the pulmonary artery carries deoxygenated blood from the right ventricle to the lungs. These exceptions are important for understanding hemodynamic monitoring (Unit 4).

- The coronary arteries supply the myocardium (heart muscle) with oxygenated blood during the resting phase of the cardiac cycle (diastole). Immediately beyond the left ventricle, these arteries branch off the aorta.

  — Coronary veins carry the metabolic waste products of myocardial activity back into the venous circulation via the right atrium.

- The venous system contains approximately 60% of a person's total blood volume. This volume is hemodynamically inactive because it does not contribute directly to blood pressure and cardiac output. Interrelated physiological mechanisms utilize this venous reserve by diverting blood to selected organs to maintain optimal cardiac output.

- Miles of capillaries form a vascular network between the arteries and veins within the body tissues. At this microcirculatory level, gas ions and nutrient molecules move across the capillary membrane for cellular metabolism.

3. **Blood Components:**

- An adequate number of red blood cells and available hemoglobin for oxygen association are essential for cardiac oxygen transportation/delivery. Alterations in RBC, hematocrit (Hct), or hemoglobin (Hgb) levels can affect the adequacy of oxygen delivery.

- A situation of inadequate oxygen supply may occur when there is a low Hct and/or low Hgb value and a SaO_2 value that is WNL. In this situation, the few number of RBC's or an inadequate supply of Hgb molecules are carrying all the oxygen ions possible. This situation results in an inadequate oxygen delivery to the tissues.

4. **Age Variations:**

- Most pediatric cardiac conditions are congenital structural abnormalities or right heart dysfunction secondary to prematurity and pulmonary problems. Septal defects or malposition of the great vessels result in cardiac dysfunction early in life.

— Children rarely suffer from the effects of impaired coronary blood flow. The problems associated with CAD develop after the long standing presence of risk factors and physiological aging.

— Children experience fewer alterations in electrical impulse transmission than adults. Dysrhythmias in a child indicate major cardiac dysfunction.

• The cardiac function of healthy, elderly persons typically meets their daily activities. However, advancing years reduces the ability to withstand periods of increased cardiac workload.

— Asymptomatic valve disease and mild CAD may affect an elder's ability to withstand increased cardiac workload. Such persons suffer an increased risk of acute angina, myocardial infarction or congestive heart failure during the management of an acute episode of another medical condition.

Physiological Review:

1. Cardiac Cycle:

• Cardiac function is dependent upon: (1) electrical impulse transmission, (2) valve effectiveness, (3) pump efficiency, and (4) circulation to the heart muscle. Dysfunction of one component affects the function of another component.

• A sequence of electrical impulses transmitted through the myocardium triggers the contraction of the heart muscle. The effectiveness of this pumping action is dependent upon an adequate supply of potassium, calcium, and magnesium.

• Impulse transmission begins in the sinoatrial (S-A) node in the right atrium of the heart. It travels to the atrioventricular (A-V) node and then along the neural fibers in the ventricular wall of the heart. An electrocardiogram (ECG or EKG) is the visualization of the electrical impulse transmission.

- In response to the atrial segment of impulse transmission, the atria contract and blood flows into the ventricles. In a similar manner, the ventricles contract in response to the ventricular segment of impulse transmission. With ventricular contraction, blood flows to the lungs (from the right side of the heart) and to the periphery (from the left side of the heart).

- The cardiac valves serve as gates which open and close to augment the forward flow of blood through the chambers of the heart. Their movement synchronizes with myocardial contraction and the pressure of blood within each chambers. Auscultation of the closing of valves represents a heartbeat (lub-dub).

- The rate and force of contraction can quickly change in response to organ and tissue needs. The volume of blood pumped each minute, or the cardiac output (CO), is calculated and adjusted according to an individual's body weight (cardiac index or CI).

2. **Vascular Resistance:**

- Arteries constrict and offer varying degrees of resistance against which the heart must pump. The terms for this process are systemic vascular resistance (SVR) or afterload.

  — The degree of vasoconstriction or vasodilation may vary according to the physiological needs of different organs and tissues. Selected organs (myocardium, brain, and kidneys) receive sufficient blood supply to maintain vital physiological functions in spite of a limited total blood supply.

- Blood pressure is the wave of blood flow through the arteries which can be auscultated or recorded on monitoring equipment. The peak, or highest reading, is the systolic pressure. The lowest point, or diastolic pressure, occurs between waves when the heart is at rest. The difference between the highest and lowest reading is the pulse pressure.

Section 2: PATHOPHYSIOLOGY

A coordinated electrical impulse transmission sequence normally triggers the heart action as the master pump. Disease processes, which affect either the impulse transmission or the pumping capability, impair cardiac function. When diminished pumping ability occurs, the blood flow through the heart chambers changes. The output or forward flow diminishes and results in backup or pooling of blood in the structures entering the heart. These changes affect one or both sides of the heart. Visualization of each side of the heart as separate structures connected by the lungs (pulmonary circulation) clarifies the physiological consequences.

Tracing the Flow of Blood:

1. Venous (deoxygenated) blood enters the right atrium from the vena cava. It flows from the right atrium through the tricuspid valve into the right ventricle. The right ventricle pumps blood into the pulmonary artery and into the lungs.

   - If the right side of the heart is an ineffective pump, or the flow is obstructed through this side of the heart, the backup will occur first in the vena cava. With additional backup in the venous flow, congestion occurs in the liver, spleen, and veins of the lower extremities. Peripheral edema may occur.

   - Ineffective forward flow from the right side of the heart (pulmonary hypertension) will lead to impaired pulmonary circulation. Subsequently, altered gas exchange occurs. Retention of carbon dioxide (respiratory acidosis) and/or insufficient oxygenation (hypoxemia) may develop. The subsequent inade-

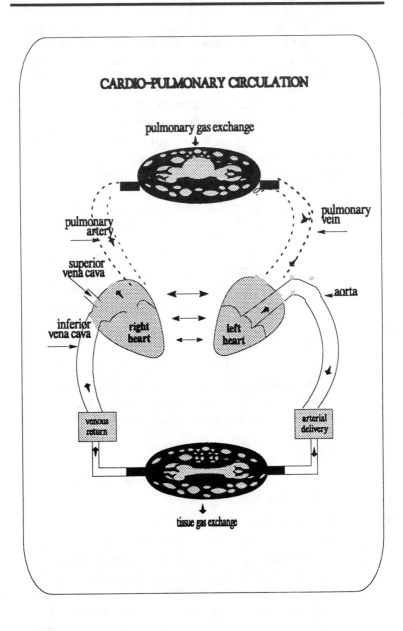

quate blood flow through the left side of the heart will lead to an inadequate flow into the general circulation.

2. Oxygenated blood flows from the lungs in the pulmonary veins and enters the left atrium of the heart. It flows from the left atrium through the mitral valve into the left ventricle. The left ventricle pumps the blood through the aortic valve and into the aorta and general circulation. Recall that during the resting phase, or between heartbeats, blood flows into the coronary arteries.

   • If the left side of the heart is an ineffective pump or the flow is obstructed flow through this side of the heart, the backup first distends the left ventricle. If this situation continues, the left ventricle muscle enlarges (hypertrophy). Aortic or mitral valve stenosis or insufficiency contributes to this clinical situation.

   — The pooling of blood may extend back up into the pulmonary veins and into the pulmonary circulation. If this situation develops quickly (pulmonary edema), it is often a medical emergency.

   — If the backup develops slowly, the pooling may extend backward into the right side of the heart and eventually lead to congestion in the venous circulation.

   • Ineffective forward flow from the left side of the heart affects the cardiac output (CO) and the adequacy of systemic and peripheral circulation. The heart initially beats faster in an attempt to pump more blood per minute into the circulation. The arteries initially constrict in an attempt to divert blood to vital body organs. If these initial compensatory measures are not effective, the blood pressure falls and vital organ function becomes impaired.

Cardiac Dysfunction

Varying disruptions in electrical impulse transmission occur when impaired functioning or death of myocardial tissue is present. An altered transmission or other atypical origins of transmission may enter the sequence. These changes impact on the effectiveness of the myocardial contraction (the pumping capacity). To minimize the irreversible damage to cardiac cells, it is essential to identify the early signs of impaired cardiac function.

1. Conditions which primarily impair impulse transmission include:

   - Abnormal serum electrolytes levels

   - Hypoxemia

   - Injured, dead, or scarred myocardial tissue

   - Drug toxicity or overdosage

   - Acid-base abnormalities

2. Conditions which primarily impair the heart's pumping ability include:

   - Infections of the myocardium or cardiac structure

   - Fluid, pus or blood within the pericardial sac

   - Diseased valves

   - Acidosis

   - Cardiomyopathy

3. Conditions which primarily impair circulation to the heart muscle include:

   - Atherosclerosis (coronary artery disease)

   - Coronary artery spasm (angina)

   - Thrombosis of a coronary artery (myocardial infarction "MI")

Section 3: DIAGNOSTIC TECHNIQUES OF CARDIAC FUNCTION

General Assessment Guidelines

- **Chest Pain:** Characteristic symptom indicative of insufficient oxygen supply to the myocardium. Using the PQRST acronym, objective and subjective characteristics are evaluated:

  — "P"= provoked by exercise or stress. What are the VS at rest and following activity? Does the chest pain awaken the person at night while sleeping?

  — "Q"= quality: throbbing, stabbing, crushing, or pressure.

  — "R"= region: isolated or radiating. Ask the person to locate the origin of the pain. Does the person use their finger (specific and localized) or his/her hand (wider area of involvement)?

  — "S"= severity: self-reporting assessment using a 1 to 10 scale with 1=minimal and 10=the most intense pain ever experienced.

  — "T"= time: frequency and duration. What did the person do to try to alleviate the pain? What was the response to the action taken?

- **Cardiac-related dyspnea:** Exertional dyspnea (breathlessness with physical activity) accompanied by a chronic, dry nonproductive cough. Is the person able to complete a sentence without pausing midsentence for deep breaths?

- **Skin color:** Pallor, peripheral, or circumoral cyanosis.

- **Systemic perfusion:** Decreased blood pressure and increased pulse rate; decreased intracranial perfusion (lethargy, confusion); decreased renal perfusion (decreased urinary output); decreased peripheral pulses; decreased venous return (peripheral edema).

Decision Tree for Acute Chest Pain

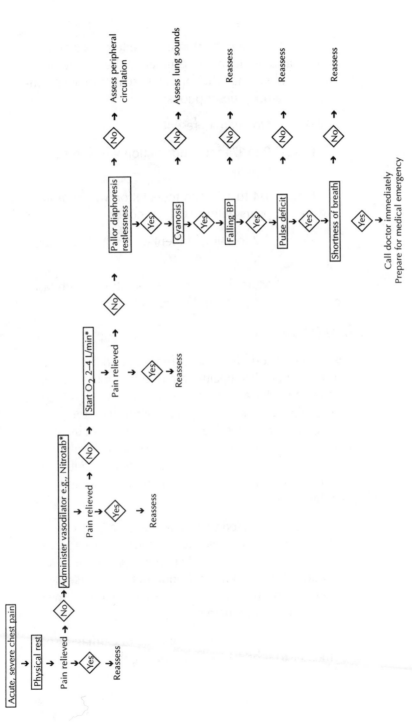

* As prescribed

- Varying finger indentation in the edematous area serves as a guideline for estimating the degree of interstitial edema. The following scale provides consistency among descriptions:

    0   No edema present

    +1   0 to 1/4 inch indentation which disappears rapidly

    +2   1/4 to 1/2 inch indentation which disappears within 10-15 seconds

    +3   1/2 to 1-inch indentation which disappears within 1-2 minutes

    +4   More than 1-inch indentation which lasts longer than 5 minutes

Heart Sounds

Assessing heart sounds involves more than determining the apical pulse rate. The health care provider must also determine the character and quality of the sounds. This technique requires practice in a quiet environment for obtaining data using a systematic approach. Focus on one sound at a time. Gaining a firm experiential foundation in hearing the basic S1 and S2 heart sounds is essential prior to seeking opportunities in recognizing unusual and abnormal sounds.

- It is recommended that the nurse gain experience with various adult age groups, various chest sizes and various heart rates. Experience with auscultating heart sounds when other equipment is in use (oxygen and/or mechanical ventilation) increases the ability to differentiate sounds.

- One may complete the sequence of cardiac assessment 1 to 4 or 4 to 1 by following the sites. Either sequence is acceptable.

Heart Sound Auscultation Sites

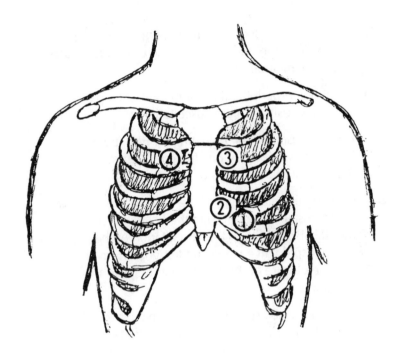

Sequence for Auscultating Heart Sounds

1. *Mitral valve area:* 5th intercostal space (5ICS)

    Midclavicular line (MCL)

2. *Tricuspid valve area:* 5th intercostal space (5ICS)

    Left lower sternal border

3. *Pulmonic valve area:* 2nd intercostal space (2ICS)

    Left sternal border (LSB)

4. *Aortic valve area:* 2nd intercostal space (2ICS)

    Right sternal border (RSB)

1. The first "lub" sound (S_1) accompanies the closure of the mitral valve between the left atrium and ventricle of the heart. It occurs with the onset of systole (ventricular contraction). The diaphragm of the stethoscope at the apex of the heart, overlying the left fifth intercostal space (5ICS) in the midclavicular line (MCL), facilitates optimal auscultation.

   • Carotid and peripheral pulsation are often palpated simultaneously with the auscultation of the S_1 sound.

   • Prior to auscultation, palpating for PMI (point of intensity) with heel of one hand of the provider also locates optimal site for auscultation.

2. Positioning the diaphragm of the stethoscope over the fifth intercostal space (5ICS) to the left lower sternal border (LLSB), facilitates the auscultation of the closure of the tricuspid valve between the right atrium and ventricle. The closure of this valve contributes to the S_1 "lub" sound.

3. The second "dub" sound (S_2) accompanies the closure of the pulmonic valve which is located between the right ventricle and the pulmonary artery. This second sound occurs with the end of systole and the beginning of diastole. The diaphragm of the stethoscope placed at the second intercostal space (2ICS) to the left of the sternal border (LSB) facilitates optimal auscultation.

4. The diaphragm of the stethoscope placed to the right of the sternal border (RSB) over the second intercostal space (2ICS) facilitates the auscultation of the closure of the aortic valve. This valve located between the left ventricle and the aorta can be heard. The closure of this valve contributes to the S_2 "dub" sound.

   • Occasionally the S_2 sound is "split" when the pulmonic and aortic valves close separately. Physiologic (normal) splitting of S_2 occurs during inspiration.

- When S_2 splitting is heard both during inspiration and expiration, an abnormality may exist. This sound is difficult to recognize with a fast heart rate.

5. After mastering the ability to accurately identify normal heart sounds, recognizing abnormal heart sounds becomes easier. There are many abnormal sounds which may indicate serious heart conditions or changes in cardiac function.

- Gallops (S_3 or S_4) are abnormal, low pitched sounds which occur during diastole and are often difficult to hear unless the heart rate is slow. However, S_3 gallops frequently occur when the heart rate is fast.

  — The S_3 occurs soon after the S_2 sound. With a relatively slow heart rate, this extra heart sound is more easily identified. It is created by resistance to ventricular filling.

  — The S_4 sound occurs immediately prior to the S_1 sound and is often referred to as an atrial gallop. Placement of the bell of the stethoscope at the apex of the heart when the person is lying on his or her left side facilitates the auscultation of a gallop. It is produced by decreased ventricular compliance or increased ventricular volume.

  — Summation gallop is the term used for the simultaneous occurrence of S_3 and S_4.

- Clicks are high-pitched sounds heard during systole when diseased or calcified valves are snapping open.

- Inflammation of the pericardial sac produces a pericardial friction rub. Placement of the diaphragm of the stethoscope at the apex and along the left sternal border facilitates the optimal auscultation of the typical scratchy, grating, rasping sound. When the person is leaning forward or exhaling, a friction rub is more audible.

- Murmurs are turbulent blood flow through the heart and large vessels. They may occur at various points during the cardiac cycle depending upon which valves are not closing adequately. The sound varies in quality, intensity, and pitch.

CARDIAC MONITORING

Bedside monitoring of cardiac impulse transmission is an important aspect of high acuity cardiovascular nursing care. The bedside nurse is valuable in the recognition of the onset of changes and trends in cardiovascular status and response to specific nursing interventions and medical therapies.

For the nurse beginning to practice high acuity cardiovascular nursing care, cardiac monitoring may appear as a monumental challenge. The presence of multiple wires to the patient and the possibility of dysrhythmias often seem overwhelming. An extension, elaboration, and refinement of the assessment of pulse rates and heart sounds provide the basis for this "high-tech" intervention.

Basics of Interpretation

The normal sequence of cardiac impulse transmission begins in the SA node, travels to the A-V node and then progresses along the neural fibers of the ventricular muscle wall. Myocardial contraction occurs subsequent to each segment of the electrical impulse. An EKG tracing records only the electrical impulse, not the muscle contraction.

- Normal characteristics and parameters for each component of an electrical impulse configuration include:

    — *P wave:* normally the first component; is followed by atrial contraction; typically positive deflection (atrial depolarization).

    — *PR interval:* interval of time associated with the transmission of impulse from the SA node to the A-V node; WNL: 0.12-0.20 second interval.

— *QRS complex:* interval of time associated with the transmission of impulse from the A-V node along the neural fibers of the ventricle muscle wall; it is followed by ventricular contraction and systole; complex should end on the isoelectric baseline; WNL: less than 0.12 second interval (ventricular depolarization).

— *T wave:* wave that follows the QRS complex which reflects resting ventricle (ventricular repolarization).

Guidelines for EKG Interpretation

Step 1: A quick scan of a 6-second strip often provides clues to an abnormality.

- Look for the presence of each element of each configuration: P wave, QRS complex, T wave, and the presence of any additional components.

- Are all components present in each configuration?

Step 2: Determine an estimated heart rate based on the number of P-QRS-T complexes or R-to-R intervals that occur during the 6-second interval. Then multiply that number by 10 for an estimate of the heart rate per minute. Atrial and ventricular rates are determined in a similar manner.

Step 3: Determine the presence of any deviations from normal parameters. Identify if these deviations are associated with atrial or ventricular dysfunction.

- If a deviation in the regularity of P-QRS-T configurations is noted, and the QRS complex is WNL, then the dysrhythmia is probably atrial in origin.

- If a deviation in the regularity of P-QRS-T configurations is noted, and the appearance or interval of the QRS is abnormal, then the dysrhythmia is probably ventricular in origin. Prompt identification of these dysrhythmias and appropriate initiation of resuscitation efforts avert sudden death situations.

- Junctional dysrhythmias are often more difficult for a novice to recognize. Typically, the QRS is WNL but the rate, location, or appearance of the P wave is altered.

Step 4: Interpreting a given tracing includes naming the basic or underlying rhythm as well as the additional alteration or superimposed dysrhythmia. Often a combination of rhythms is present. For example: sinus rhythm with 3 PAC.

Step 5: Identify the physiological effect that this cardiac rhythm or dysrhythmia is having on the individual. As changes in cardiac activity impact upon the effectiveness of myocardial contractility, cardiac output, and systemic perfusion, the physiological response influences subsequent nursing and/or medical intervention.

Placement of Leads

The exact placement of leads (electrodes) is not as crucial for monitoring cardiac rhythms as it is for diagnosis of disease states (12-lead EKG). The most important aspect of electrode placement for monitoring is identifying the location that provides clear configuration with minimal interference from noncardiac electrical activity (artifact).

Cardiac monitoring typically involves the placement of 3-5 electrodes to the chest. Two electrodes provide a recording between the points of attachment with the third electrode providing a grounding function. The preferred electrode placements are modifications of the standard 12-lead ECG which is used for diagnostic purposes.

1. **Lead II.** The placement of the positive (+) electrode is lateral to the apex of the heart (point of maximum impulse) with the negative (-) electrode placed on the right upper anterior thorax below the clavicle. The placement of the ground electrode is on the upper left anterior thorax or below the right pectoral muscle. This popular placement provides positive deflections for all complexes with prominent QRS.

Placement of Monitoring Lead II

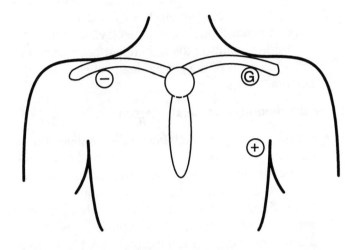

Simulated EKG tracing in Lead II
NOTE: With different placement leads, normal deflection are:

Positive

Negative

Biphasic

- When noncardiac (artifact) electrical transmission is recorded on the EKG tracing or monitor, try an alternative placement of the positive lead. For example, less artifact is noted with mechanically ventilated persons when the positive electrode is placed on the left upper anterior thorax below the clavicle. The negative electrode remains in the right upper anterior thorax. The placement of the ground lead is below either pectoral muscle.

2. **Troubleshooting Inadequate Recording:**

   - Each lead produces a characteristic configuration in relation to the baseline (isometric line). Configurations may be positive (deflections above the baseline), negative (deflections below the baseline), or biphasic (deflections above and below the baseline). If the appropriate configuration is not present, check the placement of the leads. If the placement is appropriate, then an underlying pathological condition may be present which warrants further investigation.

   - Other muscle activity (body movement, seizure, shivering) or bedside electrical equipment may produce atypical waveforms on EKG tracing or on the monitor.

   - Increasing the amplitude on the monitor enlarges a small size of cardiac impulse tracing.

   - When the skin surface beneath the electrodes is clean and dry with minimal diaphoresis, the quality of the tracing is optimal quality. Excess body hair may interfere with optimal skin-electrode contact. An adequate amount of moist conductive gel provides good contact between the electrode and skin surfaces. Usually electrodes are replaced daily but may require more frequent changing.

   - Incisions, insertion sites for central lines or dressings, may occur at optimal electrode placement sites. Changing the lead or placement of electrodes is acceptable. No single lead placement is appropriate for every person and clinical situation.

Interpretation of Common Rhythm Patterns

1. Sinus Rhythm:

- **Normal sinus rhythm (NSR)** refers to a normal P-QRS-T configuration within a given time interval. The rate of each configuration is the same as the heart rate. For adults, 60-100 beats/minute is WNL.

    — Parameters are appropriate for age differences. For example, a child of 3 years has a normal heart rate of 80-110 beats/minute (bpm). Thus, an EKG with normal configuration and a rate of 100 bpm exhibits NSR appropriate for age. This same rate is fast or tachycardiac for a 48-year-old person on quiet bedrest or sleeping.

- **Sinus bradycardia** refers to normal P-QRS-T configurations that occur more slowly than expected within a given time interval. Rate: < 60 beats/minute for an adult. This alteration is common for a person's current decreased level of activity or for athletes in peak physical conditioning.

    — Slow heart rate may produce clinical problems if the heart rate is unable to increase in response to increased physical activity or increased cellular metabolic needs. Inadequate perfusion of oxygen and nutrients to the periphery may occur with a slow heart rate.

    — When a seriously slow heart rate persists and systemic perfusion is decreased (hypotension, decreased LOC), a CODE or cardiac arrest may occur. (Refer to Unit 1: "Concepts Common to High Acuity Nursing Care" for additional information on resuscitation.)

    — When a seriously slow heart rate recurs, triggering impulse transmission may require artificial stimulation (pacemaker) to maintain a heart rate WNL. (Refer to later section in this unit for additional information on pacemakers.)

- **Sinus tachycardia** refers to normal configurations that occur regularly and more quickly than expected within a given time interval. The alteration is common for a person with increased level of activity or cellular metabolic needs. Rate: > 100 beats/minute for an adult.

  — If prolonged, fast heart rates produce clinical problems due to an associated increased workload on the myocardium. A shortened resting time (diastole) between ventricular contractions affects the perfusion of the myocardium.

  — Hypotension and angina may accompany increased rate. Bedrest (reduced physical activity) reduces cellular metabolic needs. Supplemental oxygen usually minimizes anginal symptoms.

Normal Sinus Rhythm

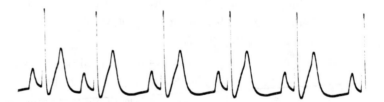

Sinus Bradycardia

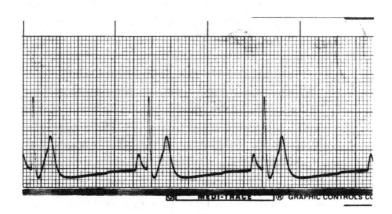

Sinus Tachycardia

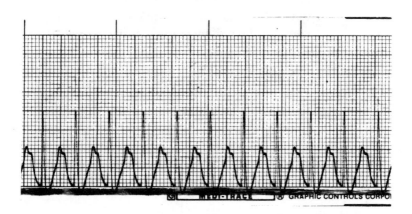

2. Atrial Dysrhythmias:

- Atrial tachycardia occurs when more S-A node stimulations occur than A-V node triggering. The rate of P waves is faster than the number of QRS complexes. In many cases, an irritable area in the atrium fires repetitively at a rate of 150-250 times a minute. The AV node blocks many of these impulses to prevent a fast ventricular rate. QRS complexes are WNL and occur at regular, fast intervals. The description of paroxysmal atrial tachycardia (PAT) is an abrupt onset and cessation of atrial tachycardia.

  — Accompanying clinical manifestations are related to altered circulation: palpitations, lightheadedness, angina, fainting (syncope).

  — Unilateral carotid sinus stimulation, Valsalva, exhaling against a closed glottis, straining to defecate, or vomiting may precipitate conversion to NSR. Identification and treatment of the underlying cause minimize recurrence.

  — Prolonged, fast heart rates increase cardiac cellular metabolism. Thus, impaired coronary circulation and myocardial ischemia may result (angina) when this type of increased cardiac workload occurs.

  Atrial fibrillation (A-fib) occurs when there are rapid, chaotic atrial impulses generated at exceedingly fast rates with irregular A-V and ventricular conduction. QRS complexes are WNL but occur at irregular intervals because the AV node acts as a filter to prevent a fast ventricular rate. Emboli often form in quivering atria and travel in the pulmonary or systemic circulation.

  — A pulse deficit is typical when the apical rate is faster than the radial rate. Variability in audible blood pressure readings is common. Other symptoms relate to altered perfusion.

— Pharmacological management with digoxin, calcium channel blocking agents, quinidine, or procainamide usually controls symptoms. When indicated, electrical cardioversion disrupts persistent, chaotic atrial activity.

— The risk of this dysrhythmia increases with infective cardiac disease (endocarditis), following cardiac surgery, and with valvular heart disease.

• **Premature atrial contractions (PAC)** occur when the triggering of the P-QRS-T sequence originates from a source other than the S-A node within the atrium. The P-QRS-T sequence occurs early and a compensatory pause follows. The configuration of each component is WNL, but the heart rate is irregular.

— A person may experience a sensation within the chest (the feeling that the heart has "skipped a beat"). A series of PAC's often produce an irregularity in pulse or heart sounds. Typically, PAC's interrupt an underlying sinus rhythm.

— PAC's are usually untreated unless they accompany other cardiac problems. Common causes include:

• Electrolyte imbalances

• Hypoxia

• Stimulants: Nicotine, Caffeine, Theophylline

• After gaining expertise with the above described atrial dysrhythmias, the nurse should also learn to recognize the following additional atrial dysrhythmias.

— Sinus pause

— Atrial flutter

— Sick sinus syndrome

— Sinus block

— Wandering atrial pacemaker

Atrial Fibrillation

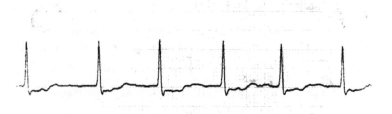

Sinus Rhythm with PAC

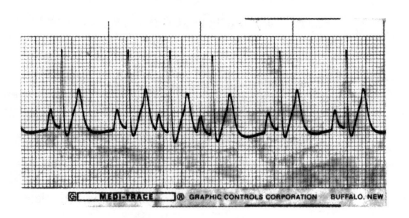

3. Junctional Dysrhythmias:

- These dysrhythmias occur when the S-A node fails to initiate impulse transmission and the A-V junction "fires" instead. This response is a protective mechanism to ensure basic/intrinsic cardiac function. Without S-A node triggering, the intrinsic/default junctional rate is only 40-60 bpm.

- Independent junctional impulses spread upward to the atria and downward along the ventricular fibers.

  — QRS complexes and T waves appear normal in configuration.

  — An inverted atrial depolarization (P wave) occurs in lead II. Altered timing includes: (1) P wave precedes the QRS but with a shortened PR interval, (2) P wave may be buried within the QRS and not be identifiable, or (3) P wave may follow the QRS complex.

- Accelerated junctional rhythms are 60-100 bpm and junctional tachycardia produces rates greater than 100 bpm.

- Although these dysrhythmias occur in healthy adults, they typically accompany heart disease or drug toxicity.

  — With this dysrhythmia, altered cardiac output occurs due to changes in heart rate. Observe the effects on systemic perfusion.

- After gaining expertise with interpreting the above described junctional dysrhythmias, the nurse should also learn to recognize the following additional junctional dysrhythmias:

  — Premature junctional contractions (PJC)

  — Junctional tachycardia

4. Heart Block (atrioventricular block):

- This group of dysrhythmias involves alterations in the impulse conduction sequence which result in various delays along the pathway. Due to the varying types of conduction delays, an associated bradycardia exists. Impaired impulse conduction often decreases the heart's ability to increase the rate and force of contraction when cellular need increases.

- **First degree heart block** occurs when the impulse transmission through the A-V node delays momentarily producing a PR interval that is consistently greater than 0.20 seconds. As there is no delay in conduction along the ventricular pathway, the QRS complex has normal configuration. The R to R interval is regular but lengthened. Clinically, this dysrhythmia is asymptomatic and is detected on EKG.

  — This dysrhythmia resembles sinus rhythm but the PR interval is lengthened. It may not require treatment if the person is asymptomatic and cardiac activity can adapt to changes in physical activity. Lightheadedness, angina, or dyspnea may develop if the heart rate decreases and cardiac output diminishes.

First Degree Heart Block

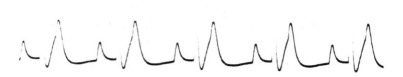

- **Second degree heart block** occurs with the presence of a prolonged PR interval and some atrial impulses not transmitted through the A-V node. As some P waves are not followed by a QRS complex, an irregular heart rate occurs. When indicated, atropine or pacemaker insertion restores an adequate heart rate.

  — As some impulses from the atria to the ventricles are periodically blocked, irregular heart rate occurs. Atrial rate is faster than the ventricular rate.

  — **Mobitz type I** (Wenckebach) occurs in recurrent cycles in which the PR interval progressively lengthens until an impulse is completely blocked at the A-V node. The QRS complex is WNL. The atrial rate is regular but the ventricular rate is irregular. This dysrhythmia is often transient and may resolve spontaneously.

  — **Mobitz type II** occurs when the PR interval is constant but some P waves are not followed by a QRS complex. A regular or irregular pattern of blocked P waves (or dropped QRS complexes) is identified. More severe bradycardia and diminished cardiac output results. This dysrhythmia occurs with severe cardiac ischemia or MI. It often progresses to more serious heart block.

Second Degree Heart Block

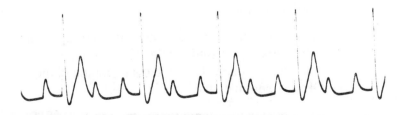

- **Third degree A-V heart block** (complete heart block) occurs when the PR interval varies and the QRS complexes widen. P waves do not consistently precede each QRS complex. As profound bradycardia results, restoration of adequate cardiac activity usually requires pacemaker insertion. The ventricular rate usually is 20-40 (beats/minute.) There is no relationship between the P and QRS complexes. Each chamber (atria and ventricle) acts independently of one another.

- After gaining expertise with interpreting heart blocks, recognizing bundle branch blocks is suggested.

Third Degree Heart Block

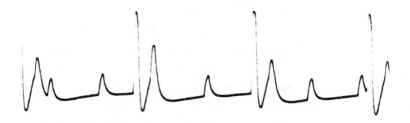

5. Ventricular Dysrhythmias:

- These dysrhythmias are often life-threatening and require immediate intervention when cardiac output is seriously impaired.

- **Premature ventricular contractions** (PVC) are usually triggered by a ventricular ectopic source other than the A-V node. Thus, the configuration of the QRS is abnormal, wide, and bizarre.

  — Cardiac output diminishes with each PVC. Hemodynamic changes occur with each PVC.

— May occur in patterns: coupled or paired (periodic occurrence of two consecutive PVC's); bigeminy (one PVC with one normal QRS); trigeminy (2 normal QRS followed by 1 PVC).

— Unifocal PVC's produce similar abnormal configurations; whereas, multifocal PVC's produce varying abnormal configurations. Multifocal PVC's typically originate from a variety of sites.

— Certain clinical considerations warrant close observation for the pattern of PVC's. Frequent PVC occurrence may develop into more serious ventricular dysrhythmias. Therefore, most coronary care units have protocols for the administration of IV lidocaine when one or more of the following situations occur:

- More than 6 PVC's per minute

- PVC's occurring together (couplet pattern)

- Multifocal PVC's

- A run of ventricular tachycardia (more than 3 consecutive PVC's in a row)

Premature Ventricular Contractions (PVC)

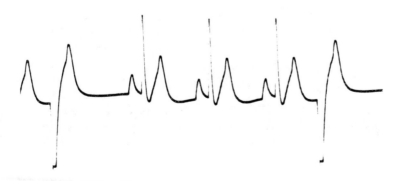

- **Ventricular tachycardia (V-tach)** refers to a run of 3 or more consecutive PVC's. As cardiac output progressively decreases or V-tach continues, this dysrhythmia usually leads to a CODE situation.

  — Indications for the placement of an automatic defibrillator (AICD) implant include persons at risk for recurrent runs of PVC's, recurrent V-tach or survivors of sudden cardiac death. A sensor continuously monitors cardiac rhythm. The AICD delivers an electrical countershock within 15-20 seconds of the onset of ventricular tachydysrythmia.

Ventricular Tachycardia (V-tach)

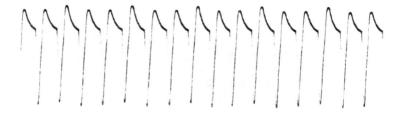

- **Ventricular fibrillation (V-fib)** occurs in response to numerous ectopic impulses which cause rapid stimulation and ventricular quivering. As there is no identifiable rhythm or cardiac output with this dysrhythmia, this is always a CODE situation.

- After gaining expertise with interpreting the above described ventricular dysrhythmias, recognizing the following dysrhythmias is suggested.

  — Torsades de Pointes

  — Agonal beats

— Pulseless electrical activity (PEA) formerly termed electromechanical dissociation (EMD)

Ventricular Fibrillation (V-fib)

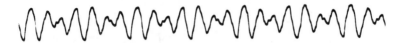

6. Paced Rhythms:

- A pacemaker produces an artificial stimulation of a cardiac impulse. This stimulation may trigger an atrial impulse and/or a ventricular impulse. A characteristic spike occurs on an EKG tracing when the pacemaker delivers an impulse.

- "Captured paced beat" refers to the paced stimulation which triggers the appropriate impulse. "Failure to capture" refers to the absence of a subsequent cardiac impulse. This loss of "atrial kick" and filling of the ventricles may lead to hypotension.

- The timing of paced beats is typically on a "demand cycle" which produces a stimulation only when the interval following an intrinsic impulse exceeds given parameters. With the refinement of the pacemaker and other electrical equipment construction, there is minimal risk of interference in pacemaker functioning from certain equipment (microwave).

- The temporary insertion of a pacemaker may occur following cardiac surgery or when severe cardiac ischemia is present. Recurrent, severe bradycardia is an indicator for the insertion of a permanent pacemaker.

Atrial and Ventricular Paced Rhythm

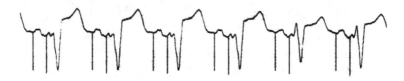

Measures to Optimize Cardiac Function

1. Cardiac Catheterization:

- This diagnostic test provides visualization of the coronary arteries when coronary artery disease (CAD) or an intracardiac condition is suspected.

  — Assessment of right heart function is possible by threading a catheter toward the heart through the femoral vein. Assessment of O_2 saturation levels determines the presence of left-to-right shunting. Obtaining right ventricular and right pulmonary artery (PA) pressures provides data about pulmonary vascular pressures.

  — Assessment of left heart function is possible by threading a catheter toward the heart through the femoral artery and aorta. Entrance into the coronary arteries, which are just above the aortic valve, occurs during diastole when the aortic valve is closed.

- *Pre-Cath Care includes:*

  — Adequate explanation of the procedure and activities; baseline anticoagulation status; chest x-ray; serum electrolytes; signed consent; pre-medication and NPO.

  — Determine shellfish and iodine allergy history as reaction is possible.

- *During Cath Care includes:*

  — Person may experience chest pain when dye is inserted. The risk of dysrhythmias increases as altered coronary circulation occurs during this procedure.

  — Person is asked to cough to elevate intrathoracic pressure and thereby increase the flow of dye into the coronary arteries. Most persons experience warm to burning sensation and the urge to urinate when the dye is injected.

- *Post-Cath Care includes:*

  — Flat in bed for 12-24 hours. Pressure at the insertion site is expected if femoral approach is used. As the size of the catheter and vessel is large, there is risk for bleeding from the insertion site or into the retroperitoneal space. Post-op routine for VS and assessment of insertion site are required. No flexion of involved extremity, especially at the hip, is permitted. Sand bags and pressure dressing at insertion site minimize hematoma formation.

  — Peripheral pulse assessment is essential as this procedure involves major vessels. Compare findings with pre-cath baseline and with opposite extremity. The following acronym is a helpful guideline ("NAVY"):

    - "N"—neural function distal to insertion site: numbness, tingling, pain.

- "A"—arterial function distal to insertion site: pallor, mottled appearance, decreased peripheral pulses, cold skin temperature, poor capillary return.

- "V"—venous function distal to insertion site: dark reddened appearance, sensation of fullness, tissue edema.

- "Y"—inguinal area assessment for bleeding at insertion site.

— Cardiac monitoring is indicated as there is the risk for dysrhythmias within the first few hours following this procedure.

2. **Medications:**

- Digitalis preparations (example: lanoxin, digitoxin) increase the force of contraction and slow the heart rate.

- Vasodilators (example: nipride, nitroglycerin, morphine sulfate) decrease the workload of the heart by dilating the vessels or decreasing the systemic vascular resistance.

- Analgesia (example: morphine sulfate) decreases the perception of pain, relieves anxiety and the stress response, and decreases the workload of the heart by producing vasodilation.

- Supplemental oxygen ensures an adequate supply to the myocardium and minimizes sporadic dysrhythmias due to myocardial irritability (example: PVC, PAC).

- Electrolyte replacement ensures optimal electrical impulse transmission and contractility: magnesium, potassium, calcium.

- Anticoagulant therapy minimizes the extension of an existing clot formation and minimizes the formation of new clots. Heparin is usually initiated first with continuous infusion dosages adjusted to maintain therapeutic PTT levels. Oral preparations are initiated before heparin is discontinued. Refer to Unit 2, "pulmonary embolus" for additional information.

- Calcium Channel Blockers such as nifedipine (Procardia), and diltiazem (Cardizem) block the ability of calcium ions to initiate smooth muscle contraction. Resulting vasodilation increases coronary and systemic blood flow and the workload of the heart decreases.

- Beta Blockers such as propranolol (Inderal), metoprolol (Lopressor), atenolol (Tenormin) decrease the heart rate, myocardial contractility, and myocardial oxygen consumption by blocking the receptors of the sympathetic nervous system's (epinephrine) response to physiological or psychological stress.

3. **Coronary Angioplasty** or percutaneous transluminal coronary angioplasty (PTCA):

- This procedure introduces a balloon-tipped catheter into the femoral artery which is advanced upward in the aorta and then into the coronary artery. At the point of atherosclerotic narrowing, the inflated balloon compresses the plaque against the arterial wall. The lumen of the artery increases and blood flow improves. PTCA during an acute MI restores blood flow to ischemic myocardial tissue.

  — Rapid restoration of blood flow may precipitate ventricular dysrhythmias.

  — Approximately 5-10% of PTCA cases require emergency coronary artery by-pass surgery because of acute coronary occlusion.

- While the balloon is inflated, disrupted flow of oxygenated blood may precipitate varying degrees of angina. Infusing heparinized solution during this procedure minimizes concurrent thrombosis formation.

- The care following this procedure is similar to cardiac catheterization. Re-occlusion within 24 hours occurs in 25% of the cases and typically 60% reocclude within 6 months.

- Atherectomy is a relatively new procedure used in conjunction with PTCA to remove the plaque from the walls of an occluded coronary artery.

4. **Cardiac Surgery** ("open heart" surgery)

- Coronary artery by-pass graft (CAB or CABG) provides a surgical alternative for myocardial circulation around atherosclerotic and markedly narrowed coronary arteries. The use of segments from either the saphenous vein or mammary artery provides revascularization. The criteria for surgical selection currently have no age limits and include "new" or "fresh" MI victims.

   — Reports state that more than 80% of grafts remain patent 4 years after surgery. Most persons experience improved quality of life with increased physical activity, decreased incidence and severity of anginal attacks.

- Valve replacement typically involves the mitral and/or aortic valves; thus, the function of the left side of the heart is affected. Involvement of the tricuspid valve (right heart) is less common.

   — During the post-operative period, atrial fibrillation with periodic bradycardiac episodes is likely to occur. This dysrhythmia increases the potential of emboli formation from the left ventricle.

   — Auscultation of the closing of a prosthetic valve produces a distinct metallic "click."

   — Long-term anticoagulant therapy minimizes the potential thrombosis formation around the prosthesis. Prophylactic antibiotic therapy administered prior to invasive treatments and dental procedures minimizes bacterial colonization around the prosthetic site and subsequent complications from endocarditis.

- Optimal systemic perfusion occurs during CAB or value replacement procedures by heparinizing the person's blood, diverting it from the heart for oxygenation, and pumping it back into general circulation. The heart is free of blood flowing through its chambers during the surgery. Iced saline solution placed inside the heart produces a localized hypothermia and protects myocardial tissue from the effects of hypoxia.

- *Post-Op Care includes:*

  — Person will be intubated for 12-24 hours or until ABG's are stable. The placement of 1-3 chest tubes is typical — two pleural and one mediastinal. As the mediastinal tube is not placed in the pleural space, it does not fluctuate with respiratory activity.

  — Re-establishing optimal hemodynamic status varies according to pre-operative status and the number of by-pass grafts. The degree of left myocardial hypertrophy and dilatation also affects post-operatively hemodynamics. Refer to Unit 4 for additional information on hemodynamic monitoring.

  — The risk of dysrhythmias is greatest during the first 12-48 hours. Optimal myocardial response occurs when serum electrolytes (especially magnesium, potassium, calcium) and ABG's are maintained WNL. Identifying trends in cardiac enzymes is essential as there is a risk of MI occurring during and immediately after surgery.

5. **Intra-aortic balloon pump (IABP):**

- This temporary invasive procedure involves the placement of an inflatable balloon catheter into the upper portion of the descending aorta via femoral arterial insertion site.

— The timing of the inflation/deflation of the balloon is synchronized with ventricular contraction. When the balloon inflates during diastole, blood moves into the coronary arteries and further down the arterial system. The balloon deflates when the aortic valve opens and the left ventricle contracts. Thus, the exodus of blood from the heart flows easily into the relative void created by the deflated balloon. Cardiac workload is diminished until cardiac function is restored.

Section 4: EXAMPLES OF COMMON CLINICAL CONDITIONS

Myocardial Infarction (MI)

Sudden occlusion of a coronary artery causes the cessation of oxygenated blood flow to the myocardium beyond the obstructed vessel. Cellular damage occurs within 20 minutes following occluded blood flow. Irreversible damage occurs if occlusion lasts longer than 6 hours: hypoxic cells die. As a consequence, the death of a portion of the heart muscle interferes with electrical impulse transmission which may precipitate potentially lethal ventricular dysrhythmias.

Approximately half of MI deaths occur during the first 1-2 hours following the onset of pain. Unfortunately, the majority of persons delay seeking medical attention for 1-4 hours following the onset of pain. Many persons die before reaching the hospital and the majority of in-hospital deaths occur within the first 24 hours. Dysrhythmias precipitate sudden cardiac death.

The common age of occurrence for the first MI is 45-64 years. Underlying atherosclerosis is present in coronary arteries and also in arteries of other organs. The good news is that there is a 70-80% survival rate for the first MI.

Poor prognosis is associated with age greater than 80 years, previous MI, or presence of chronic respiratory disease or uncontrolled diabetes mellitus.

1. Pathophysiology:

- As cardiac cells and the myocardium are metabolically very active and have no storage capability for oxygen and nutrients, signs of ischemia develop within 8-10 seconds of decreased arterial blood flow. Within 20 minutes, signs of cellular damage appear. Tissue injury is reversible if blood supply is restored within 4-6 hours. The area surrounding the affected area becomes inflamed causing secondary ischemia and impaired function. This area recovers with restored blood flow.

  — While irreversibly damaged myocardium can heal with scar formation, impaired cellular function is often permanent. Impaired impulse transmission and effectiveness of myocardial contraction often results.

- Most MI's occur in the coronary artery which supplies the left ventricle. Thus, cardiac output decreases and backup into the pulmonary circulation develops. The risk of cardiogenic shock and pulmonary edema increases proportionately with the myocardial damage.

- Following the occlusion of an artery, the smaller secondary connecting branches progressively assume the task of providing adequate circulation around the occluded segment. These smaller vessels require time to build up the strength of their walls or become "conditioned" for the increased flow and intravascular pressure. Collateral circulation is another term for this secondary circulatory mechanism. It continues to develop throughout convalescence and cardiac rehabilitation.

2. Indications:

- Characteristic pattern of intense, "crushing" chest pain that is not relieved by rest or nitroglycerin tablets, and lasts longer than 15 minutes. It often radiates to the left arm, neck, or shoulder.

  — Accompanying symptoms include:

    - Nausea

    - Anxiety

    - Dyspnea

  — Among the elderly, the pain manifestation is often less dramatic. Fainting and profound weakness may be the only symptoms indicating sudden diminished cardiac function and subsequent fall in cardiac output into the general circulation.

  — Persistent hiccoughs may accompany an inferior MI.

  — Characteristic EKG changes: elevation of the ST segment with peaked or inverted T wave.

  — Serum CPK with MB bands and LDH isoenzyme elevate producing characteristic patterns.

3. Medical and Nursing Management:

- Initiation of thrombolytic therapy within the first 6 hours of the onset of pain can restore myocardial circulation (reperfusion) by dissolving the recent clot formation. The following agents may be used: streptokinase, urokinase, tissue-plasminogen activator (tPa) or acylated plasminogen streptokinase activator complex (APSAC).

  — Established protocols determine the criteria for administration and treatment procedures. For example, the administration of tPa requires a large bore peripheral line (not a central line).

— History of recent surgery, TIA, CVA or GI bleeding tendencies may contraindicate thrombolytic therapy.

— Successful reperfusion includes a return of the EKG to WNL; relief of chest pain and early peak/decrease in CPK-MB enzymes levels. There also is a risk for reperfusion ventricular dysrhythmias.

• Care measures during an acute MI focus on decreasing cardiac workload and preserving aerobic cellular metabolism:

— Bedrest in position of comfort to promote physical rest and decrease the cardiac workload

— Pain control with liberal doses of morphine sulfate

— Oxygen therapy to minimize tissue hypoxia

— EKG monitoring for early detection and treatment of dysrhythmias

— Stool softeners to decrease constipation and bradycardia from straining

— IV nitroglycerin to dilate coronary arteries and promote coronary perfusion (may also cause severe headaches and/or hypotension)

— IV heparin to prevent the extension of an existing coronary thrombosis. Dosages are titrated (adjusted) to maintain therapeutic PTT or ACT values.

• Recognize the early signs of complications:

— Cardiogenic shock. This complication is more likely to develop when the occlusion affects the perfusion resulting in damage to the left ventricle. The clinical signs of diminished forward blood flow from the left ventricle results in decreased systemic perfusion.

— Pulmonary edema. This complication is more likely to develop when perfusion to the left ventricle occurs. The backup of blood flow through the left ventricle extends back into the pulmonary vascular system.

— Dysrhythmias. Disrupted impulse transmission often occurs with injured cardiac tissue. With myocardial ventricular involvement, dysrhythmias occur and prompt treatment is essential. Delayed impulse transmission often results in heart blocks or bradycardia which may require an artificial pacemaker to trigger a normal rate.

— Approximately 95% of all persons with an MI will have dysrhythmias; some may be potentially lethal. And, approximately 40% will experience bradycardia that may warrant corrective treatment.

— Reocclusion or secondary MI may occur in 5-10% of cases during the early recovery period. This complication manifests with recurrence of characteristic symptoms, recurrent EKG changes, and a rise in CPK-MB.

— Rupture of the chordae tendineae or papillary muscles. These structures normally provide optimal opening and closure of the mitral and tricuspid valves. With papillary muscle attachment involvement, impaired valve movement produces an inadequate flow through the heart chambers and into general circulation. Left-sided heart failure and/or cardiogenic shock may develop.

Focused Bedside Assessment

The following guideline provides data expected from a head-to-toe assessment of an individual experiencing an acute cardiac dysfunction. Acute MI leading to left side heart failure is used as an example. No other pathophysiological problem involving other body systems is included.

- **General Appearance:** "severe chest pain" usually radiating to the back, neck, jaw, or left arm; restlessness; anxiousness; feeling that something very wrong is happening; sitting upright (orthopneic); cold diaphoresis; pallor

- **Level of Consciousness:** oriented but agitated or impatient; hyper-alert; confused if elderly

- **Head and Neck:** initially findings are WNL; signs of right CHF appear later as backup effects of left failure progresses; jugular vein distention (JVD) is a late symptom (considerable pulmonary congestion is present before this symptom appears)

- **Cardiac Status:** initial tachycardia with an onset of ectopic beats; diminished S_1; onset of S_3 and/or S_4; systolic murmur may develop; normotensive progressing to hypotensive; characteristic elevation of ST segment and inverted T wave on EKG

- **Respiratory Status:** tachypnea; increasing presence of adventitious sounds in lower lobes; increasing presence of crackles and wheezes; nonproductive cough progresses to frothy sputum production

- **Abdomen:** nausea and/or vomiting; BS present but decrease in frequency and intensity; soft with no tenderness

- **Urinary Elimination:** adequate but decreasing in volume; clear appearance

- **Extremities:** decreasing intensity of peripheral pulses and slowing of capillary refill; increasing pallor and decreasing skin temperature; feet and hands may begin to appear mottled

- When the person is turned on his/her side, the nurse assesses similar respiratory sounds and similar skin manifestations

If additional data is observed, a more detailed assessment of the involved system is required; additional areas of physiological dysfunction may be present and confound the present cardiac problem.

Congestive Heart Failure (CHF)

Heart failure is a state in which the heart is no longer able to pump sufficient quantities of blood to appropriate structures to meet the metabolic needs. Thus, heart failure is pump failure resulting in congestion or pooling of blood within either or both sides of the heart. This circulatory overload through the heart has forward (output) as well as backup (input) consequences.

This secondary condition stems from an underlying pathophysiological problem. Several factors influence the development of this condition.

1. Pathophysiology:

- One major factor contributing to the development of CHF is preload or the amount of blood in the heart chambers before contraction occurs. Conditions that influence preload include:

  — Valves do not open or close adequately, thus allowing blood to remain or return to the chambers.

  — Tachycardia does not allow time for sufficient emptying and filling of the heart chambers.

  — Septal defects allow blood to flow from one side of the heart to the other side with decreasing amounts being pumped out into general circulation.

  — Dysrhythmias do not permit sufficient emptying of the chambers.

  — Intravascular fluid overload requires an increase in the heart rate to move the added volume through the heart chambers.

  — Damaged/diseased myocardium does not contract strongly enough to fully empty its chambers.

- A second major factor contributing to the development of CHF is afterload or the resistance which the heart must pump against in order to push blood from its chambers. Conditions that influence afterload include:

  — Increased systemic vascular resistance (SVR) or hypertension

  — Pulmonary hypertension due to chronic pulmonary disease (cor pulmonale)

  — Valvular stenosis which creates a barrier against which the heart must pump to push blood into circulation

- Other factors affecting the development of CHF include:

  — Anemia which reduces the oxygen carrying capacity and causes tachycardia as a compensatory response

  — Increased cellular metabolism which increases the cellular need for oxygen and the removal of metabolic waste products; tachycardia will occur as a compensatory mechanism

  — Increase or decrease in blood volume which affects cardiac rate; in an attempt to circulate whatever blood volume is available, the heart rate initially increases when hypovolemia, shock, or hemorrhage is present

  — Parenchymal disease of the myocardium; i.e., cardiomyopathy

2. Indications:

The characteristics of CHF can be divided into left- or right-sided failure and are described in terms of forward (output) and backup (input) aspects. In this manner, a care provider can identify specific clinical manifestations exhibited by individuals and understand the rationale for selected interventions. The evaluation of intervention effectiveness relates to the resolution of clinical manifestations specific to the side of the heart involved.

- Left-sided heart failure is typically an acute condition that has a rapid onset.

  — Forward (output) effects relate to diminished cardiac output; onset may be gradual or abrupt; cerebral hypoxia, restlessness, confusion, bad dreams; decreased blood pressure; decreased urinary output in the daytime and nocturia at night.

  — Backup (input) effects relate to congestion extending into the lungs: dyspnea with physical activity; fatigue and muscle weakness; nonproductive cough progressing to frothy sputum; orthopnea and paroxysmal nocturnal dyspnea (PND); onset of S_3 or S_4; increasing pulmonary artery/capillary wedge pressures.

- Right-sided heart failure typically is a chronic condition that has a slow, gradual onset.

  — Forward (output) effects related to diminished circulation to the lungs leading to impaired gas exchange: underlying pulmonary vascular hypertension; borderline, normal ABG values.

  — Backup (input) effects relate to venous congestion extending back into systemic organs: liver enlargement leading to RUQ pain; possible ascites which often raises the diaphragm and impairs breathing; anorexia; venous congestion leading to dependent, pitting edema; weight gain; nocturia; PND; increasing central venous pressure; jugular vein distention (JVD).

3. Medical and Nursing Management:

- Interventions to improve cardiac pump effectiveness include the following medications:

  — Cardiac glycosides (digitalis, digitoxin) increase the force of contraction and slow the cardiac rate.

— Dopamine in low doses promotes vasodilation to major organs to ensure adequate perfusion. Dobutamine improves cardiac contractility.

— Diuretics reduce fluid overload thereby reducing preload.

— Vasodilators reduce afterload. For example, angiotensin converting enzymes inhibitors (ACE inhibitors) suppress the renin-angiotensin-aldosterone cycle and its vasoconstricting and Na+ retaining actions.

- When indicated, a variety of medications modify the pathophysiological effects. It is essential to closely monitor for adverse and interacting effects. Altered electrolyte levels commonly develop.

- Identifying and managing the underlying causative factors minimize the development and progression of this condition.

Cardiac Tamponade

A sudden accumulation of blood or fluid in the pericardial sac which surrounds the heart may be a life-threatening event.

1. Pathophysiology:

- Since the pericardium can stretch only minimally, an accumulation of 20+ ml will compress the heart and impair cardiac function. Cardiac filling during diastole and outflow during systole (cardiac output/CO) progressively decreases.

2. Indications:

- This condition often is a cardiac emergency when it occurs following cardiac surgery or blunt chest trauma. The myocardium is weakened and often is not capable of withstanding this additional physiological stressor of surgery or trauma.

- Clinical manifestations relate to diminishing cardiac function: tachycardia with thready pulse; dyspnea; falling BP leading to confusion and/or restlessness; decreasing urinary output; pallor with cold/clammy skin.

  — Increased heart rate is an early compensatory mechanism which attempts to move limited blood supply within the heart chambers into general circulation. This mechanism only temporarily produces a sufficient cardiac output. Decreased CI with tachycardia is an indicator of cardiac failure.

  — The onset of clinical manifestations may develop rapidly especially if cardiac tamponade occurs following cardiac surgery.

- Physical assessment findings:

  — Muffled heart sounds due to listening through accumulated fluid

  — Elevated central venous pressure (CVP > 12 mmHg) due to backup of blood in the venous system before entering the right chambers of the heart

  — Pulsus paradoxus (fall of > 10 mmHg in systolic BP during inspiration) due to blood pooling in the pulmonary veins during inspiration

  — Narrowing pulse pressure: the difference between the systolic blood pressure reading and the diastolic reading progressively narrows

  — Enlarged mediastinum on chest x-ray

3. Medical and Nursing Management:

- Pericardiocentesis is the insertion of a needle into the pericardial sac to drain excess fluid accumulation. This medical procedure may be done at the bedside.

- Creating a surgical window in the pericardium and the placement of mediastinal chest tube are corrective measures.

- Providing adequate fluid replacement increases the cardiac filling pressures, cardiac output, and blood pressure. (Refer to Unit 4: "Hemodynamic Monitoring" for assessment guidelines reflective of intravascular volume.)

Pericarditis

This is an acute or chronic inflammatory process involving the surface of the heart and surrounding membrane (pericardium). It involves an acute or chronic dry irritation when associated with fluid accumulation within the pericardial sac (effusion).

1. Pathophysiology:

- Other cardiac and systemic conditions such as acute MI, chest trauma, and cardiac surgery often accompany this clinical condition. Pericarditis may also occur with the following systemic conditions: uremia, rheumatic disease, malignancy, or radiation therapy.

- Effusion (fluid accumulation) within the pericardial sac may accompany the inflammatory process. The pericardium progressively becomes thick and fibrous. Consequently, it progressively constricts and compresses the heart preventing adequate filling and emptying of the heart chambers. This process progresses without spontaneous reversal of symptoms.

2. Indications:

- Chest pain is typical, but the description may vary. It is often increased by supine position and with a deep breath. Rapid, shallow breathing usually minimizes the severity of pain.

- Associated symptoms in right ventricular failure are dyspnea, fatigue, and fever.

  — With increased venous backup: distended neck veins, ascites, and leg edema occur.

  — Decreased flow to the left side of the heart leads to decreased cardiac output which causes fatigue on exertion, dyspnea, and delayed capillary refill.

- *Friction rub:* The diaphragm of the stethoscope placed at the left lower sternal border (LLSB) or apex (PMI) while the person is sitting upright and leaning forward facilitates optimal auscultation. A grating, creaking sound is heard with each heartbeat.

- Atrial dysrhythmias may occur during the acute phase. Hemodynamic findings often reflect altered circulation through the heart chambers when associated effusion occurs.

- Elevated cardiac enzymes (CPK, LDH) occur during the acute phase, but elevations are not characteristic of an acute MI. ASO titer may be elevated and indicate an associated immunologic disease.

3. **Medical and Nursing Management:**

- Bedrest until fever subsides

- Nonsteroidal anti-inflammatory medication (Indomethacin)

- Pericardiocentesis if effusion is also present

- A pericardiectomy may be performed to relieve restriction from adhesions because of recurrent effusions

Infective Endocarditis

The presence of bacteria, viruses, fungi or rickettsiae circulating in the blood may colonize in the natural pockets located around the heart valves. The resultant infection affects the innermost layer of the heart (endocardium). Associated platelet fibrin thrombus occurs and supports the organism growth (vegetation).

1. **Pathophysiology:**

   - The causative organisms enter the body through any body orifice. Colonization is more common on the mitral and aortic valves than the tricuspid valve in the right heart. As prosthetic valves also have a predilection for colonization, it is important that these at-risk individuals receive prophylactic antibiotics prior to any dental or invasive procedure.

   - Vegetative emboli may occur. As the structures of the left side of heart are involved, emboli travel from the left ventricle to the brain (CVA), kidney (renal infarction) and periphery (arterial occlusion).

2. **Indications:**

   - During the acute infective stage: unexplained fever, diaphoresis, fatigue, joint pain; severity of symptoms varies

   - Classic findings:

     — Small red streaks on the fingernails and toenails

     — Painless, small hemorrhagic lesions and subcutaneous nodules in the soft tissue of the fingers, toes, nose, or earlobes

     — Retinal hemorrhages

   - Murmur characteristic of specific valve involvement

   - Presence of S_3 and S_4 heart sounds

3. Medical and Nursing Management:

- Appropriate antibiotic therapy for 6-8 weeks

- Fluid replacement and pharmacotherapy to maintain optimal hemodynamics

Cardiomyopathy

A specific cause of this heart muscle disorder is unknown (idiopathic). A wide variety of inflammatory, infective, metabolic, toxic, and genetic factors are attributed to some cases.

- Abnormalities of the valves, coronary arteries or pulmonary disorder are not characteristic—only the myocardium is involved. Ventricular changes determine the classification: dilated (congestive), hypertrophic (muscle enlargement), or restrictive.

- Medical therapies, including pharmacotherapeutics, initially control symptoms and the progression of myocardial dysfunction.

  — If these measures are ineffective and no other concurrent medical problem (co-morbidity) is present, the person may be a candidate for cardiac transplantation. Evaluation for eligibility is a detailed process and does not guarantee that a transplant will be available in time. (Refer to Unit 1 for additional information on organ procurement and transplantation.)

  — The mean life expectancy of a person waiting for cardiac transplantation is 3 months. Mechanical devices are temporary and used when end-stage cardiac failure is present, and no suitable donor is immediately available.

Valve Disease

Dysfunctional heart valves most frequently involve the mitral and aortic valves which affect optimal left-sided heart function. Thickening of the valve leaflets and adhesions of the chordae tendineae result in a reduction in the size of the valve opening. Impaired forward flow of blood is progressive.

1. Pathophysiology:

- Most cases develop subsequent to a streptococcal infection (rheumatic fever). Clinical manifestations may not develop until later in life when increased cardiac workload is required.

  — Pregnancy may precipitate valvular dysfunction as a normal 50% increase in blood volume occurs. Circulating this added volume provides added strain on the valves which may not adequately close. This valvular insufficiency requires added ventricular contractibility to move the blood into circulation. If the left ventricle is unable to compensate for the valve insufficiency, left ventricular failure and pulmonary edema may result.

- Nonrheumatic causes are related to staphylococcal endocarditis, drug abuse, autoimmune diseases, or degenerative changes among the elderly.

2. Indications:

- The CO is WNL while at rest but decreases with exertion.

- Dyspnea, fatigue, palpitations and nonproductive cough are typical and accentuate with physical activity.

  — Paroxysmal nocturnal dyspnea (PND) occurs when the person assumes a recumbent position especially when sleeping at night. Blood shifts from the trunk and lower extremities into the venous system returning to the heart, thereby increasing the workload of the right heart. The sudden increase in pulmonary congestion causes the person to wake up with acute breathlessness 2-4 hours after going to bed. Sitting upright with feet dependent relieves this symptom.

3. Medical and Nursing Interventions:

- Surgical replacement of the damaged valve(s) is the most effective treatment. Post-operative care is similar to coronary by-pass procedures. There is a risk for atrial fibrillation and the possibility of secondary emboli formation following valve replacement.

  — Persons over 40 years of age are at greater risk for atrial fibrillation.

- Long-term anticoagulant therapy is required to minimize thrombus formation on the prosthesis.

Unit 4

Care of Individuals with High Acuity Circulatory Conditions

This unit addresses a variety of high acuity circulatory conditions associated with varying degrees of impaired circulation and altered perfusion to systemic organs. Persons with these conditions were traditionally cared for in critical care units. However, as the trends in health care delivery shift to ambulatory, extended, and home health settings, the principles of high acuity nursing care and related nursing interventions will extend beyond the walls of the traditional acute care hospital.

The information presented in this unit focuses on circulation and perfusion. It builds upon the understanding of effective cardiac function as the master pump.

Section 1: REVIEW & OVERVIEW

Anatomical Review

An adequate circulatory system delivers sufficient amounts of oxygen and cellular nutrients to the tissues. The venous system carries metabolic waste products to the lungs or kidneys for elimination. In order for this process to be effective, the interaction among three components is essential. The heart functions as a master pump. The vessels constrict and dilate to ensure optimal blood flow throughout the system, and sufficient quantities of red blood cells and hemoglobin serve as the major oxygen ion transporters.

Physiological Review

1. In a balanced physiological state (homeostasis), some body organs require more metabolic supplies than others. The heart requires approximately 5-7% of the cardiac output. The brain requires approximately 15%, and the kidneys require approximately 21%. The lungs, intestinal tract, abdominal organs, skeletal muscles, and peripheral skin of the extremities utilize the remaining 60%.

   • The myocardium receives only 5-7% of the systolic cardiac output and more than 70% during diastole. The heart has high metabolic needs and minimal storage capability. Therefore, it extracts approximately 75% of the oxygen and nutrients from every ml delivered.

2. Total blood volume for an average sized adult is 5.5 liters. The heart rate and stroke volume (SV) provide the basis for calculating the amount of blood pumped from the heart or cardiac output (CO). Stroke volume refers to the amount of blood ejected with each heart beat.

   • *Cardiac Index*—Cardiac output (CO) value typically is adjusted according to an individual's size, and body weight provides the basis for individualized adjustment of the CO.

- Ejection Fraction—The left ventricle does not eject all of the blood with each contraction. Typically it pumps 70-75% of the blood within the ventricular chamber with each contraction. Cardiac index (CI) refers to this adjustment. The left ventricle does not eject all of the blood with each contraction. Typically, it pumps 70-75% of the blood within the ventricular chamber with each contraction. Therefore, determining the amount actually ejected provides additional data about pump effectiveness within the context of understanding perfusion.

3. The vascular system contains the blood volume. Arteries typically hold 15%, capillaries hold 15%, and veins hold 70%. Due to the ability of arteries and capillaries to dilate and constrict, blood actively moves through the vascular system. Blood movement back to the heart through the veins is more passive. Skeletal muscle contraction provides a milking action against the veins to facilitate the forward movement of venous   blood toward the heart, and valves prevent backward flow of blood due to gravity.

   - The heart and vessels respond to the metabolic needs of tissues and organs. To deliver needed metabolic supplies, the heart beats faster, and the arteries and capillaries dilate. As a result, there is increased blood movement throughout the system.

      — The circulatory response to increased physical activity is an example of physiological adjustment to meet cellular metabolic need. This response is typically experienced by an individual who is walking fast, climbing stairs, or experiencing a fever. When the physiological need is met, the heart rate and vasodilation return to baseline values.

Section 2: PATHOPHYSIOLOGY

When the heart is unable to circulate blood and adequately perfuse tissues, a state of shock exists. Decreased tissue perfusion results in widespread impaired cellular metabolism. Any factor that alters cardiac function, blood volume, and blood pressure contributes to the development and progression of a shock state. Unless compensatory mechanisms or interventions reverse the process, shock from any cause progresses to organ failure and ultimately to death.

1. The underlying cause and/or the intravascular volume status determine the classifications of shock.

- Underlying physiological causes of shock include:

  — Systemic infection (sepsis or septic shock)

  — Severe allergic response (anaphylactic shock)

  — Loss of blood or plasma (hemorrhagic or hypovolemic shock)

  — Profound anemia or carbon monoxide poisoning (transport shock)

  — Heart failure (cardiogenic shock)

  — Vasodilation below the level of spinal cord injury (neurogenic shock)

  — Mechanical barriers to blood flow such as pulmonary embolism, cardiac tamponade, tension pneumothorax (obstructive shock)

- Intravascular volume status related to a shock state is either hypovolemic or normovolemic.

  — Hypovolemic shock occurs when a loss of blood or plasma results in a decrease in intravascular volume. Shifts in fluid from the intravascular compartment to the interstitial compartment also lead to hypovolemic shock.

  — In addition to hemorrhage, conditions which trigger fluid shifts and hypovolemia include: dehydration, burns, nephrotic syndrome, and pancreatitis.

- With normovolemic shock, there is no change in intravascular volume; however, the capillary space holds a disproportionate amount of intravascular volume. An associated loss of vascular tone leads to massive vasodilation. The descriptive terms "distributive" and "vasogenic" also refer to normovolemic shock.

  — Conditions which produce an imbalance between the amount of blood available within the intravascular compartment and the size of the capillary space include: anaphylactic, neurogenic, and septic shock.

  — With septic shock, there also is an increase in capillary permeability secondary to lactic acidosis. A release of bradykinin accenutates the vasodilation and often accelerates the progression of shock.

2. Regardless of the physiological cause or the altered intravascular volume, all types of shock produce a similar sequence of pathophysiological events. The blood and plasma do not circulate throughout the vascular system in a timely manner. There is delayed or diminished venous return to the heart. Cardiac output diminishes and all tissues, in turn, suffer from the effects of inadequate perfusion.

   - In all types of shock, cells are either not receiving an adequate supply of oxygen or are unable to use the available oxygen supply.

     — Inadequate oxygen delivery develops when low cardiac output, insufficient numbers of red blood cells, or inadequate intravascular volume occur.

     — Factors which impair cellular use of oxygen include: cellular swelling, interstitial fluid excess, activated clotting sequence, and inflammation of cells adjacent to damaged ones.

— Monitoring oxygen delivery (SaO_2 and paO_2) and oxygen utilization (SvO_2) are essential to detecting an early change in cellular metabolic need. Appropriate interventions ensure adequate oxygen delivery and conserve oxygen utilization while the underlying cause is corrected. (Refer to Unit 2: Care of Individuals with High Acuity Respiratory Conditions for additional information.)

• In a similar manner, impaired glucose use relates to either impaired glucose delivery or impaired uptake by the cells. Alterations in glucose metabolism include: fever, bacteria, vasoactive toxins, endotoxins, histamine, and kinins. Hyperglycemia and insulin resistence also develop.

— The cellular need for energy sources is often greater than available glycogen resources. Depletion of stored fat and glycogen occurs within a few hours of increased cellular need. Protein sources are then used for energy instead of maintaining cellular structure, function, and repair. The risk of organ failure increases as the protein resources decrease.

3. Early compensatory response:

• The sympathetic nervous system responds first to decreased cardiac output. The baroreceptors in the carotid sinus and aortic arch detect a fall in blood pressure which produces the release of epinephrine and norepinephrine. Subsequently, there is an increase in heart rate, cardiac output, myocardial contractility, and arterial vasoconstriction.

• These initial responses circulate the available blood supply and restore (or maintain) an adequate blood pressure. Identifying and correcting the underlying cause restore perfusion before impaired tissue and cellular metabolism develops.

4. Second or decompensated stage:

- When blood pressure and cardiac output continue to fall and the early responses are ineffective, decreased perfusion to the heart, brain, and kidneys triggers a secondary compensatory response. The limited blood supply in general circulation is now directed to the heart, brain, and kidneys to maintain life sustaining and vital physiological functions.

- Vasoconstriction and decreased blood supply to other tissues and organs (skin, intestinal tract, and skeletal muscles) provide a sufficient supply of blood to the vital organs. This "borrowing" mechanism is only effective temporarily. Restoration of an adequate blood and intravascular volume ensures optimal circulation/perfusion to the tissues.

- The renin-angiotension-aldosterone (RAA) cycle facilitates this compensatory stage to restore/maintain blood volume and blood pressure.

 — Decreased blood flow to the kidneys triggers the conversion of angiotensin in the liver to angiotensin I which is converted to Angiotensin II by angiotensin converting enzyme (ACE) in the lungs. The release of renin, a potent vasoconstrictor, triggers the conversion of angiotensin I to angiotensin II in the lungs. The presence of angiotensin II stimulates the adrenal glands to release aldosterone. The kidneys retain sodium ions and, in turn, water molecules. In this manner, restoration of intravascular volume and blood pressure occurs.

Renin-angiotensin-aldosterone cycle

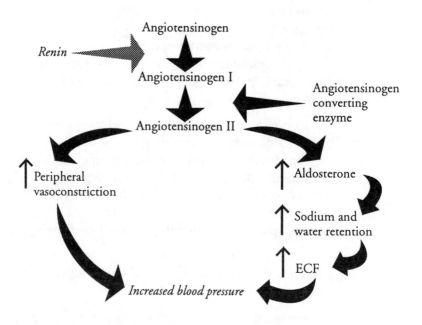

5. Late or refractory stage of shock:

- As decreased perfusion becomes more profound and lasts longer, tissue ischemia and hypoxia develop. Cellular metabolism converts from an aerobic to anaerobic state. The waste products of anaeorbic metabolism include lactic and pyruvic acids.

- The accumulation of these acids leads to lactic acidosis. Relaxation of capillary tone and increased capillary permeability occur. Capillary vasodilation increases and leads to prolonged capillary blood flow or "pooling." Fluid movement between the capillaries and the adjacent interstitial space increases the development of interstitial fluid excess or third spacing.

- Altered cellular metabolism progresses. Adenosine triphosphate (ATP) becomes the energy source for cellular function. Changes within the cell structure occur and the affected cells begin to retain fluid and swell. Cellular damage occurs, and some cells may rupture.

- As shock progresses, the systemic circulation and microcirculation no longer work in unison. Systemic vasoconstriction continues with progressive oxygen/nutrient delivery impairment. At the same time, the microcirculation continues to dilate. Venous return declines leading to decreased circulation of reoxygenated blood. A vicious cycle begins.

- Progressive ischemia of the gastrointestinal tract triggers the release of myocardial depressant factor (MDF). Decreased myocardial contractility leads to declining CO, CI, and SV values. The state of shock worsens.

- The events become progressively more severe with increasing body system involvement. A cycle develops leading to a cascading "falling domino" response. Eventually circulation and cellular metabolism are totally disrupted. All body organs and tissues become affected by impaired perfusion and hypoxia. When multiple system organ failure (MSOF) develops, there is a high mortality rate.

- The challenge of management is to: (1) replace fluid requirements, (2) support compensatory mechanisms, (3) promptly identify and correct the underlying cause, and (4) prevent organ system failure.

SECTION 3: DIAGNOSTIC TECHNIQUES OF PERFUSION

General Assessment Guidelines

1. Altered Cerebral Perfusion

- A change in level of consciousness (LOC) is due to a decrease in cardiac output (CO) or an interruption in arterial blood flow to the brain. When the systolic blood pressure falls below 60 mmHg, cerebral blood flow diminishes sufficiently to produce clinical symptoms.

- Subtle changes include: decreased wakefulness, lethargy, confusion, forgetfulness, syncope (fainting spells). Sudden changes include: severe headache, seizures, loss of consciousness.

2. Altered Renal Perfusion

- The volume of urinary output decreases in response to diminishing CO. A decreased blood supply initiates two responses: (1) vasoconstriction within the renal system and (2) triggering of the renin-angiotensin-aldosterone (RAA) cycle. Both of these compensatory mechanisms affect the filtration and reabsorption within the renal system. In response the kidneys retain fluid, and the urinary output diminishes. (Refer to Section 2 for additional discussion on the RAA cycle.)

- Early indicator: decreasing urinary output inspite of an adequate fluid intake. For an adult, urinary output that falls below 50 cc/hr warrants further assessment. A fall below 30 ml/hr may impair renal function and require prompt corrective treatment.

3. Altered Circulatory Perfusion

- Chest pain (angina) is due to a decreased amount of arterial (oxygenated) blood entering the coronary system. When the heart rate is very fast, the length of diastole may not be sufficient to permit adequate flow into the coronary arteries.

- Peripheral edema is an indicator of impaired venous return or movement of blood through the chambers of the heart. (Refer to Unit 3 for additional information on edema assessment.)

- Assessment of blood pressure and pulse provides a baseline for evaluating responses to interventions. When peripheral vasoconstriction and diminished CO are present, obtaining peripheral pulses may require a Doppler to amplify the sound of low flow states.

- A resting pulse rate above 110 bpm in an adult warrants further perfusion assessment for other supporting findings. An increased heart rate is an early physiological response to decreasing CO. The heart attempts to circulate a limited blood supply by pumping faster.

4. Altered Peripheral Perfusion

- Peripheral vascular changes occur in response to changes in CO. Peripheral vasoconstriction accompanies the early compensatory mechanism to divert blood flow from the periphery to systemic organs which perform vital functions (heart, brain, and kidneys). Assessment of capillary return is a more accurate measurement of peripheral perfusion than the temperature and color of the skin.

- The vasoconstrictive response often accentuates pre-existing peripheral diminished blood flow. With severely impaired peripheral blood flow, the tips of fingers and/or toes remain blanched. These digits may become black and gangrenous if occluded capillaries occur.

- Systolic blood pressure below 60 mmHg or the diastolic pressure above 90 mmHg are indicators of impaired perfusion.

5. Age-related assessment of perfusion

- The elderly typically have delayed capillary return as compared to middle-aged adults and children. It is not uncommon that an elder over age 62 with an adequate cardiac output also has a capillary refill of 4 seconds. Therefore, evaluation of capillary return data in context with other supporting perfusion assessment is essential.

- Young children exhibit the following general appearance ("looks bad") associated with inadequate perfusion: pale mucosa; mottled skin color; central fever with cool extremities; irritability; limp body posture; poor feeding.

Hemodynamic Monitoring

Data on the blood flow through the heart provide health care personnel with information on the adequacy of systemic perfusion. Invasive devices provide data about intracardiac pressures and central blood pressure.

Assessment by Pulmonary Artery Catheterization

1. General information

- A 4-5 lumen pulmonary catheter is one device used to measure pressures in the right side of the heart and to indirectly estimate the pressures in the left side of the heart. These pressures provide an estimate of intravascular volume and movement of blood through the heart and lungs.

- A 110 cm catheter inserted and threaded into the venous system typically enters the subclavian vein to the right side of the heart and pulmonary artery. Specific readings and trends in data include central venous pressure (CVP), pulmonary artery pressure (PAP), pulmonary capillary wedge, or occlusion pressure (PCWP or PCOP), and cardiac output (CO).

When a fiberoptic lumen is included with the catheter, continuous SvO_2 monitoring is possible.

- The complications from pulmonary artery catheter use are less severe than with the use of direct monitoring devices of left heart function. The following complications, however, may develop: dysrhythmias, sepsis, clotting, catheter kinks or knotting, pulmonary ischemia or emboli.

2. Insertion & Care Concerns

- The insertion of a PA catheter typically occurs at the bedside using sterile technique. As it is an invasive procedure, informed consent is required. When the subclavian vein is the insertion site, there is a risk of an inadvertent penetration of the pleura and subsequent pneumothorax. Chest x-ray verifies placement. Care of the insertion site minimizes the development of infections.

- Gravity flow infusion maintains the patency of fluid filled lumens. Infusion of 3 cc/hr of heparinized solution maintains the patency of the monitoring lines. Medication and IV fluid therapy are permissible through the infusion and injectate ports. Only one port is not used for any infusion: the balloon inflation port which usually has an attached syringe.

- Placement of the transducer at the level of the atrium (4th ICS, MAL) provides an accurate recording of waveforms. A change in body position or the level of the bed requires readjustment of the transducer level.

3. Central Venous Pressure (CVP)

- A CVP reading reflects the filling pressure (or preload) to the right side of the heart. Since there are no valves at the entrance to the right heart, there is minimal difference between the systolic, diastolic, and mean pressures within the right atrium and vena cava. RAP and CVP readings are normally very similar.

— A CVP reading is often interpreted as an estimate of intravascular fluid volume. This is possible because a CVP reading reflects the pressure within the great veins which hold 60% of the blood volume. A CVP reading higher than normal parameters often indicates fluid volume overload and warrants additional assessment. A CVP reading lower than normal parameters suggests fluid volume deficit and warrants additional assessment.

• Normally, there is an inter-relationship among the central venous pressure, arterial blood pressure, and urinary output. A decrease/increase in one reading accompanies a corresponding decrease/increase in the other readings. As a clinical example, an increase in the filling pressure to the right heart (CVP) typically provides an increase in the cardiac output and systemic blood pressure.

• CVP value of 0-6 mmHg typically reflects optimal right side preload and adequate intravascular fluid volume. However, some clinical situations require higher CVP values to maintain desirable circulatory function.

4. Pulmonary Artery Pressure (PAP)

• PA pressures include systolic and diastolic readings. The systolic pressure occurs with right ventricle contraction and after the opening of the pulmonic valve. The waveform associated with PA systolic pressure is a steep rise which gradually decreases as the blood flows from the ventricle into the pulmonary circulation.

• Normal PA systolic/diastolic pressures are: 15-25/5-15 mmHg with a mean PA pressure < 20 mmHg. Higher values accompany pulmonary hypertension or secondary left heart dysfunction. A dicrotic notch on the declining waveform reflects the closure of the pulmonic valve. High tidal volume and PEEP may produce atypical waveforms.

5. Pulmonary Capillary Wedge (or Occlusion) Pressure (PCWP or PCOP)

- Obtaining this reading provides an indirect assessment of left heart function. The left ventricular end diastolic pressure (LVEDP) is the amount of blood volume (and pressure) within the left ventricle during diastole and just prior to left ventricular contraction.

- To obtain this reading, the tiny balloon located adjacent to the tip of the catheter is inflated. The blood flow from the right pulmonary artery carries the balloon on the tip of the catheter into the pulmonary circulation. The inflated balloon temporarily wedges or occludes a small pulmonary arteriole. At this time, the sensor distal to the inflated balloon on the catheter tip obtains a pressure reading. This reading reflects the left atrial pressure as it backs up against the sensor. While this vessel is temporarily occluded, the pressures from the right heart chambers are not influencing these pressure readings.

  — Under normal physiological conditions, there is little difference between PAP diastolic and PCWP/PCOP pressures. With left side heart failure and increased preload pressures, the PCWP/PCOP pressures increase. Conditions associated with elevated PCWP/PCOP include: mitral &/or aortic valve dysfunction, constrictive pericarditis, volume overload, and high PEEP ventilation.

- Deflating the wedge/occlusive balloon after obtaining a reading is imperative. An inflated balloon prevents the flow of oxygenated blood through this arteriole leading to localized pulmonary ischemia or infarction.

- Normal PCWP/PCOP values are: 4-12 mmHg. Pulmonary vascular congestion begins with values > 18-20 mmHg. Pulmonary edema values > 30 mmHg.

— When PCWP/PCOP values are below normal, interventions focus on increasing intravascular volume. With elevated values, interventions focus on decreasing volume within cardio-pulmonary structures (dilators, diuretics) and increasing myocardial contractility (cardiac glycosides).

6. Cardiac Output (CO)

- Heart rate and stroke volume affect cardiac output. CI is an adjusted CO according to a given body weight and size. Other factors affecting CO include: the amount of blood volume ejected with each contraction (preload or filling), and the amount of resistance that the ventricle must pump against (afterload or emptying). High systolic blood pressure typically accompanies high systemic vascular resistance (SVR).

  — Stroke volume (SV) refers to the volume of blood pumped into circulation with each heart beat. Normal SV = 60-80 cc.

  — Ejection fraction refers to the percent of blood volume ejected with each ventricular contraction. Normal ejection fraction = 70%. MUGA is a non-invasive procedure which calculates ejection fraction.

- Change in heart rate is the greatest factor affecting CO. For healthy persons, increasing the heart rate increases the cardiac output. For persons with cardiac disease, increasing the heart rate decreases CO because of the decreasing filling time. Interventions to maintain a balance between heart rate and cardiac output focus on keeping the heart rate slow by controlling pain, anxiety, fever, hypovolemia, anemia, and hypertension.

- Thermodilution is one method for determining cardiac output. This procedure involves injecting a pre-determined bolus of cold fluid into the right atrium through the proximal lumen. The thermistor sensor at the tip of the catheter detects the change in the temperature of the blood as it passes through the pulmonary vessels. The difference between the fluid temperature at injection site and sensor is computed and converted to a numerical value on a monitor screen.

• Normal CO for an adult is: 4-8 L/min and a normal CI is 1.5-4 L/min.

Typical NSR EKG Tracing
with Associated A-line waveforms

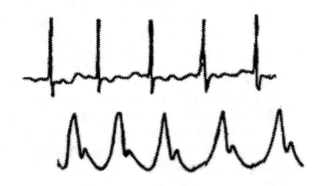

Typical NSR with PVC
with Associated A-line waveforms

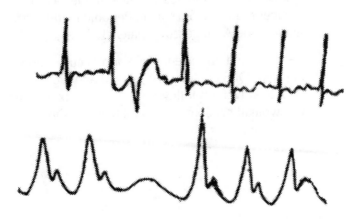

Other perfusion monitoring devices

1. Intra-arterial pressure monitoring (A-line)

- When intravascular volume and cardiac output are unstable, continuous monitoring of intra-arterial pressure provides more accurate data than auscultating peripheral blood pressures. This technique obtains systolic, diastolic, and mean arterial   pressures (MAP). The CO and MAP readings provide the data for calculating the systemic vascular resistance (SVR).

  — MAP is an estimate of SVR. Increased MAP occurs with increased SVR.

- Insertion sites include: radial artery, brachial artery, or femoral artery. Assessing for an adequate arterial blood flow distal to the insertion prior to and during the insertion of an A-line is essential.

- A rapid rise in the A-line waveform follows each QRS complex and the ventricular contraction. The highest point of the waveform corresponds to the systolic pressure. As the pressure within the ventricle falls, the waveform decreases. A dicrotic notch appears when the aortic valve closes. The lowest point or baseline is the diastolic pressure.

- The wave of intra-arterial blood flow is converted to a numerical value with the use of a transducer placed at the level of the atrium (MAL). If body position or the level of the bed changes, the level of the transducer requires adjustment. Periodic manual flushing of the A-line ensures patency.

  — A typical and consistent waveform occurs following each QRS complex. An altered and typically smaller waveform follows a PVC complex. Altered CO typically accompanies an atypical A-line waveform.

- Maintaining patency of A-lines is more problematic than maintaining patency of central venous lines. Arterial monitoring requires a high pressure system because an IV drip by gravity is not sufficient to ensure flow and prevent blood from backing up in the line. A-line requires a pressure bag setup with continuous heparinized flush of 2-5 ml/hr.

  — Blood samples for ABG analysis are obtained cautiously from this line, as there is risk of air emboli. Medications and fluid therapy are not administered through this line.

- Periodic assessment of the auscultated peripheral blood pressure provides comparative data. As circulation returns to a normal state, A-line (central) and auscultated peripheral blood pressures are within 10 mmHg.

2. Left Atrial Pressures (LAP)

- A left arterial pressure catheter (LAP) directly assesses pressures within the left side of the heart. These pressures are obtained during a cardiac catheterization and sometimes during the immediate post-operative period following open heart surgery. There is increased risk for ventricular dysrhythmias with the placement of these lines.

- LAP findings provide earlier indications of left heart dysfunction as compared to PCWP/PCOP.

Section 4: INTERVENTIONS TO IMPROVE PERFUSION

The management of an individual in a state of shock focuses simultaneously on the following three areas: (1) fluid replacement for the restoration of intravascular volume, (2) interventions which support compensatory mechanisms, (3) prompt identification and correction of the underlying cause, and (4) prevention of complications and organ system failure.

1. Fluid therapy:

- The goal is to replace fluid loss and restore intravascular volume via large-bore peripheral and central lines. Monitoring CVP and PCWP/PCOP values is essential to prevent fluid overload. The administration of sufficient fluid provides adequate venous return to the right heart without causing excess/back-up in the left heart.

- Fluid therapy replaces the intravascular deficit and additional volume that moved from the intravascular space to the interstitial space. About 2/3 of crystalloid solutions administered IV moves out of the vascular space and enters the interstitial space.

- Colloid solutions contain molecules typically large enough to remain within the vascular system. These solutions include plasma, plasma expanders, and blood products.

  — Fresh frozen plasma (FFP) provides clotting factors and plasma proteins. Low serum protein levels improve and the capillary osmotic pressure increases.

- Supplemental administration of calcium, potassium, and magnesium ensures optimal cellular function. With fluid replacement and resumed urinary output, hypokalemia frequently occurs.

- When hemorrhage is the primary cause of shock, the rapid administration of multiple units of type-specific packed cells is essential. Adequate oxygen delivery requires sufficient numbers of red cells and hemoglobin in circulation.

  — Administration of blood and blood products requires a separate infusion line. Medications, TPN and/or dextrose are not infused concurrently with blood or blood products.

2. Pharmacological therapy:

- Oxygen therapy is essential to maintain aerobic cellular metabolism.

- Vasoconstrictors (vasopressors) elevate systemic blood pressure to ensure minimum tissue/organ perfusion: (60-70 mmHg). Attempts to raise the BP higher with the use of vasoconstrictors may lead to ventricular dysrhythmias and decreased organ perfusion especially to the kidneys and splanchnic area. By constricting peripheral vessels, the heart beats faster which leads to increased myocardial oxygen consumption and possible heart failure.

  — Examples of commonly prescribed IV vasoconstrictors include: dopamine (Intropin), norepinephrine (Levophed), Amrinone (Inocor), and dobutamine (Dobutrex).

  — Low dose administration of dopamine produces systemic vasoconstriction (elevates BP) and vasodilation of the renal and mesenteric arteries (improves renal function).

  — Dobutamine also increases myocardial contractility and improved cardiac output.

- Vasodilators prevent the harmful effects of prolonged vasoconstriction. As the administration of vasodilators increases the diameter of vessels, the size of the intravascular space also increases. Filling the dilated vascular space requires additional fluid therapy. When the vascular space is full and venous return is adequate, vasodilation opens the arterioles to the lungs and other organs thereby improving general perfusion.

  — Examples of commonly prescribed IV vasodilators include: nitroprusside (Nipride), nitroglycerin (Tridil), morphine sulfate.

  — Close assessment of hemodynamic values determines the rate and volume of fluid administration. The goal is to achieve a minimum MAP of 70 mmHg. Abrupt, severe hypotension may develop as vessels suddenly open or increased urine production occurs.

- Antibiotics are essential when the underlying cause is an infection. When an individual has an open or contaminated wound along with hypovolemic shock, antibiotics are indicated.

- Heparin (low dose regime) prevents the development of venothrombosis and pulmonary emboli. Immobility and low capillary flow states contribute to clot formation.

- Medications improve myocardial contraction. Cardiac glycosides (digitalis) strengthen and slow the heart beat. Lidocaine decreases myocardial irritability and corrects some ventricular dysrhythmias; however, reduced myocardial contractility occurs.

- Histamine H_2-receptor antagonists and antacids inhibit or neutralize gastric acid secretion and prevent stress ulcers.

- Supplemental insulin maintains serum glucose levels within normal range. Hyperglycemia may develop during periods of high physiological stress and with the administration of high dextrose concentrations in total parenteral nutrition (TPN) solutions.

3. Interventions to support compensatory responses:

- Pain control minimizes the sympathetic (adrenergic) response and increased cellular metabolism.

- Monitoring SaO_2 and SvO_2 values during care activities and procedures guide planning, and implementing interventions which help to achieve a balance between cellular need and oxygen delivery capability. Mechanical ventilation improves impaired gas exchange and conserves energy expenditure during increased respiratory activity.

- A normothermic environment conserves cellular oxygen need. Shivering and chilling increase cellular metabolism. While the skin and extremities of most persons in shock are cold, application of external heat is avoided. Warmed peripheral vessels dilate and divert a limited blood supply away from vital organs.

- Nasogastric suction removes accumulated gastric secretions which may contribute to mucosal ulcer formation. Recall that an early response to shock is a decrease in blood supply (vasoconstriction) in the splanchnic vessels which supply the gastrointestinal tract. Decreased peristaltic activity and diminished tissue perfusion occur. Monitoring secretions for blood and acidity provides a guide for additional treatments.

- Early initiated nutritional support by enteral or parenteral routes minimizes protein catabolism or the breakdown of protein for energy. Enteral or parenteral solutions contain selected quantities of dextrose, amino acids, electrolytes, vitamins, minerals, and fat emulsions to meet individual clinical and nutritional needs.

4. Complications (indicators of multiple system failure):

- Decreased cerebral perfusion occurs when the MAP falls. Cerebral ischemia and subsequent damage to cerebral capillaries lead to fluid shifting from the cerebral vessels into the cerebral interstitial space. Swelling of neural cells then occurs.

  — Brain tissues are highly sensitive to shortages in oxygen, glucose, and accumulated carbon dioxide. Vessels respond by dilating to restore blood flow, but this response also increases intracranial volume.

  — Decreased LOC is an early indicator of altered cerebral perfusion. Signs of progressing increased intracranial pressure (IICP) are often masked by

the more dominant signs of shock. Sluggish pupillary response to light is an indicator of generalized
and progressive IICP. (Refer to Unit 5: Nursing
Care of High Acuity Intracranial Conditions for
additional information.)

• Decreased myocardial perfusion often precipitates
anginal symptoms and ischemic changes on EKG
tracings. Myocardial infarction may also occur.

— Eventually in the progressive sequence, all types
of shock exhibit decreasing CO and CI. The
release of myocardial depressant factor (MDF)
accompanies decreased blood flow through the
splanchnic vessels to the gastrointestinal
tract. Decreased myocardial contractility leads to
reduced CO, CI, and SV despite normal circulating blood volume. Deteriorating cardiac function
is one of the major causes of death in shock.
(Refer to Unit 3: Nursing Care of High Acuity
Respiratory Conditions for additional information.)

• Urinary output is a reflection of systemic blood flow.
Glomerular filtration is directly dependent upon
renal blood flow. Ischemic damaged kidneys lose
their ability to regulate fluid, electrolyte, and acid-
base balance. The ability to compensate for impaired
gas exchange diminishes. Metabolic acidosis develops.

— Acute renal failure (ARF) due to acute tubular
necrosis (ATN) usually is reversible within 10-14
days. Acute dialysis and ultrafiltration provide kidney function until shock is controlled and renal
function is restored. (Refer to Unit 6: Nursing Care
of High Acuity Renal Conditions for additional
information.)

• With circulatory insufficiency, blood flow to the
lungs is inadequate. Ischemic damaged alveoli
become edematous and fluid-filled. Diminished sur-

factant production occurs. Eventually, damaged alveoli collapse leading to progressive impaired gas exchange. ARDS develops.

— Decreasing oxygenation despite adequate oxygen therapy is an indicator of the development of ARDS. (Refer to Unit 2: Nursing Care of High Acuity Respiratory Conditions for additional information.)

• Impaired microcirculation of the gastrointestinal tract results when splanchnic vasoconstriction occurs. The intestinal mucosa becomes ischemic early in shock. Actual tissue necrosis, decreased peristalsis, and stagnation of secretions lead to mucosal ulceration. Segments of the intestinal tract may become necrotic.

— *Escherichia coli* and other micro-organisms normally are asymptomatic within the intestinal tract. Damaged mucosa permits microbial invasion into the peritoneal cavity or the circulatory system. Bacteria also release endotoxins into the general circulation which contribute to an increased capillary permeability in other organs. A localized intestinal infection leads to generalized sepsis and multiple system involvement.

— The release of MDF occurs with the impaired splanchnic circulation. Decreased cardiac failure progresses.

• An ischemic liver can no longer detoxify medications or bacterial endotoxins. The release of vasotoxic kinins contribute to generalized vasodilation. Conversion of glycogen to glucose is delayed or altered. Intrinsic factors in the clotting sequence are altered.

— Large quantities of blood normally flow through the liver. When blood flow diminishes through the liver, the risk of developing multiple microthrombi increases. Backup in this section of circulation accentuates the intestinal congestion and mucosal damage.

• "Third Spacing" develops when there is increased fluid movement from the vascular compartment into the interstitial space. This response occurs when the permeability of the capillaries increases. With markedly increased permeability, some plasma proteins also move into the interstitial space. These proteins exert oncotic/osmotic pressure and hold fluid in their presence. Therefore, the location of plasma proteins determines the location of excess fluid accumulation. Intravascular deficit and interstitial excess persists or may increase.

— Indicators of "third spacing" include: increasing body weight, peripheral edema, hypovolemia, decreasing serum albumin levels.

• DIC (disseminated intravascular coagulation) develops from a variety of clinical conditions and accompany varying stages of shock. A predisposing event activates either the extrinsic or intrinsic clotting pathway. Multiple microthrombi occur throughout the body leading to ischemia, hypoxia, and/or necrosis in the brain, liver, heart, lungs, and kidneys. Simultaneously, lysis or breaking up of developing microclots occurs. A cycle of coagulation, anticoagulation and fibrinolysis develops. Depletion of clotting factors and progressive hemorrhage occur.

— With sepsis, there is a profound capillary vasodilation and blood flow slows through the capillary circulation. Subsequently, activated clotting process and multiple microthrombi develop.

— Indicators of DIC include: abrupt onset of bleeding from any insertion site or mucosal surface;

presence of blood in any body fluid; abnormal increase in tissue bruising (ecchymosis, petechiae).

— Management of DIC includes: identification and correction of the underlying cause, continuous IV heparin and blood component replacement.

Stages of Shock

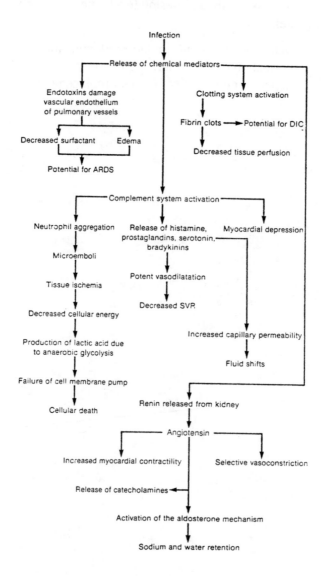

Pamela Swearingen, Marilyn Sawyer Sommers, and Kenneth Miller,
*Manual of Critical Care: Applying Nursing Diagnoses to Adult
Critical Illnesses, 2nd ed. Saint Louis: Mosby-Year Book, 1991.
Reprinted by permission.*

SECTION 5: EXAMPLES OF COMMON CLINICAL CONDITIONS

Aortic Aneurysm

This condition involves a bulging enlargement of the wall of the aorta which results from a longitudinal tear in the vessel wall. Atherosclerosis is the underlying cause for changes in this vessel wall.

1. Pathophysiology:

- The pressure of the blood flowing through the aorta separates or dissects the vessel wall at the tear site. The damaged area becomes thinner as the vessel bulges. The length of the dissection and the extent of vessel damage usually progresses and involves the coronary, subclavian, or renal arteries. Impaired perfusion to the heart, brain, or kidney may occur. With an increase in systolic blood pressure, the weakened bulging area may bleed.

- Prolonged or sudden onset of severe high pressure within the aorta causes the bulging, weakened segment of the vessel to rupture. Resulting hemorrhage is a life-threatening event and typically has a near 100% mortality rate if untreated.

2. Indications of a non-bleeding dissecting AAA (abdominal aortic aneurysm):

- Abdominal pulsation felt by the individual, usually midline, substernal region.

- Midabdominal visual or palpatable pulsations assessed by health care provider.

- Altered perfusion related to the vessel involvement (brain, heart or kidney). Blood pressure is unequal.

- Decreased perfusion distal to the aneurysm; especially sluggish capillary refill in legs.

- Chest X-ray, echocardiogram or CT scan locate the site of dissection.

3. Medical & Nursing Management:

- Hypertension controlled with medication and sedation.

- Damaged segment of the vessel is surgically replaced with a synthetic vessel graft.

Focused Bedside Assessment

The following guideline provides data associated with the second compensatory stage of shock with signs of progressive decompensation and the onset of multiple system organ failure (MSOF).

- **Level of consciousness:** decreasing LOC; agitation progressing to restlessness; confusion progressing to lethargy and unresponsiveness. *Progressive signs:* increased intracranial pressure (due to cerebral capillary permeability resulting in cerebral interstitial edema).

- **Cardiac Status:** tachycardia at rest; pulses equal bilaterally but weak & often irregular; systolic BP 30 mmHg below individual's baseline. *Progressive signs:* onset of angina; onset or increase in PVC's secondary to myocardial hypoxia; onset of S_3 and S_4 sounds; progressive myocardial depression.

- **Hemodynamic Status:** decreasing arterial and MAP pressures with narrowing pulse deficit; SVR increased; decreasing cardiac contractility (decreased ejection fraction, CO & CI). *Progressive signs:* elevating RAP/CVP, PAP & PCWP/PCOP pressures due to developing Lt. sided CHF & pulmonary edema; decreasing SvO_2 due to altered cellular metabolism.

- **Chest (respiratory) Status:** increase in adventitious sounds secondary to developing CHF; ABG's within low normal range. *Progressive signs:* increase in congested lung fields on x-ray; peripheral SaO_2 decreasing in spite of adequate oxygen therapy; progressive respiratory acidosis & hypoxia due to developing ARDS.

- **Abdominal Status:** decreased to absent bowel sounds; increased gastric acidity; initially soft but distended; bleeding from aneurysm into the peritoneal cavity results in a rigid abdomen. *Progressive signs:* taut, rigid & distended abdomen with no bowel sounds due to bleeding into peritoneal cavity, ischemic bowel or peritonitis; occult blood in gastric and intestinal secretions due to mucosal irritation.

- **Renal Status:** decreased urinary output in spite of adequate fluid intake; increased urinary specific gravity; presence of protein in urine due to renal capillary permeability. *Progressive signs:* increasing BUN and creatinine; elevating serum potassium; progressive metabolic acidosis due to developing acute tubal necrosis (ATN) or acute renal failure (ARF).

- **Extremities (peripheral circulation):** cold, clammy skin; mottled extremities; delayed capillary refill. *Progressive signs:* blackened, gangrenous digits.

- **Other Signs:** onset of oozing blood from insertion sites or mucous membranes due to onset of coagulation dysfunction or DIC; developing soft tissue pitting edema due to capillary permeability and fluid collection in interstitial space or "third spacing."

Burns

The skin is the largest organ in the human body. Its functions include protection from infection, prevention of body fluid loss, body temperature control, excretory, and secretory actions. Several factors determine a classification of a burn: (1) cause (thermal, electrical, chemical, or radiation), (2) body surface area or BSA involvement (percentage of skin damage), or depth of tissue injury (first-degree, second-degree or third-degree).

1. Pathophysiology:

- Local circulatory destruction

  — Damaged vessels occlude with cessation of blood flow. Release of histamine from damaged cells produces generalized and localized vasoconstriction. The risk of peripheral vessel thrombosis increases.

  — Intracellular, interstitial and intravascular fluid is lost from the burned tissue. Total body fluid volume decreases in relation to the area and depth of burn involvement.

  — The loss of skin integrity increases the risk of micro-organism invasion and the development of local and systemic infections. The normal flora on the skin become pathogens.

- Capilllary permeability

  — During the first 12-36 hours after a > 15% BSA burn, intravascular-to-interstitial body fluid shifts occur. This fluid contains serum proteins, electrolytes, and plasma. Hypovolemia, hemoconcentration, and increased blood viscosity develops. The risk for thrombosis formation increases.

  — The accumulation of fluid within the interstitial space produces soft tissue edema. The interstitial space can accomodate large volumes of fluid. Body cavities can also accomodate large quantities of fluid. "Third spacing" refers to the accumulation of excess fluid in atypical locations. With fluid resuscitation measures, the total fluid volume in all compartments may increase despite an intravascular deficit. An increase of 2.2 pounds of body weight equals 1000 ml of fluid excess.

— The intravascular-to-interstitial fluid shift within the lungs may alter gas exchange. The fluid shift within the kidneys may impair renal filtration and reabsorption. Within the gastrointestinal tract, the fluid shift leads to damaged mucosa.

— Damaged cells release potassium ions which pass into the vascular compartment. Hyperkalemia may develop especially if the renal dysfunction is also present.

• Capillary healing

— Within 24-48 hours after a burn, intravascular fluid loss typically ceases and excess interstitial fluid begins to move back into the intravascular compartment. This is a period of diuersis. Hemodilution of blood components and electrolytes develops. Adequate renal function usually adjusts to the increase in vascular volume by increasing the urinary output.

• Cardiovascular dysfunction

— Immediately following a burn, catecholamine secretions (epinephrine and norepinephrine) produce systemic and pulmonic vasoconstriction. However, this response cannot sustain normal blood pressure and perfusion when the circulatory volume continues to decrease.

— Following a major burn, CO may decrease to 30% of preburn level. This decrease triggers the release of MDF into circulation. Cardiac dysfunction progresses.

- Pulmonic dysfunction

  — Direct injury due to inhalation of high temperature fumes damages the naso-tracheal mucosa. The resulting burn swelling and secondary inflammatory response may obstruct the airway. An inadequate supply of oxygen to the alveoli may result.

  — Compartmental fluid shifts and pulmonic vasoconstriction alter the alveolar capillary permeability. Altered gas exchange may develop at the alveolar level of respiratory activity.

- Gastrointestinal dysfunction

  — The decrease in total intravascular volume leads to decrease in gastrointestinal perfusion. Impaired motility and intestinal ischemia develops. Ischemia increases permeability of the GI mucosa to bacteria and endotoxin invasion. The risk of sepsis increases.

- Metabolic and immunologic changes

  — Altered perfusion to cells results in altered metabolism and a hypermetabolic state occurs. Cellular oxygen consumption and caloric requirements markedly increase and often are greater than oxygen delivery capability. Typically, metabolic requirements double within 4-12 days after a burn and remain elevated until healing occurs. The presence of hypovolemia and "third spacing" accompanies a hypermetabolic state.

  — Nutrient intake and body caloric reserves often do not meet the cellular metabolic need. With the depletion of body calories/fat reserves, protein becomes the source of energy. Negative nitrogen states develop and delayed healing occurs.

  — Following a major burn, neutrophils and T-cells lose their ability to combat microorganism invasion, and the risk of systemic infection increases.

— Evaporative heat loss and hypermetabolic state contribute to the difficulty in maintaining normal body temperature.

2. Indications:

- The "rule of nines" provides a standardized estimate of the extent of a burn injury by body surface area (BSA). Using the following chart, the total percent of tissue damaged is calculated.

Rule of Nines

Body Area	Infant	Child	Adult
Head	21%	17%	9%
Chest/Trunk	18%	18%	18%
Back	18%	18%	18%
Each Arm	9%	9%	9%
Each Leg	12%	14%	18%
Genital Area	1%	1%	1%
Totals	100%	100%	100%

- Respiratory involvement: singed hairs on the head and nasal passage; swelling of naso/oral pharyngeal mucosa; crackles; stridor; severe hoarseness; altered ABG's.

- Cutaneous involvement: blisters, blebs, or dry-leathery eschar.

- Cardiovascular involvement: decreased cardiac filling (low CVP & PAP values); hypovolemia (low PCWP/PCOP, CI, CO, & BP); decreased pump effectiveness (elevated PCWP/PCOP).

- Secondary renal dysfunction: decreasing urinary output in spite of adequate fluid intake.

- Secondary gastrointestinal dysfunction: decreasing

intestinal activity progressing to loss of peristalsis and abdominal distention; increasing gastric acidity; presence of occult blood in gastric secretions or feces.

3. Medical & Nursing Management:

- Fluid resuscitation is essential to restore intravascular volume. Various formulas provide accurate parameters for the IV administration of large volumes during the initial hours. The use of adjusted formulas during the period of diuresis minimizes the risk of hypervolemia.

- When handling the affected areas sterile technique minimizes the development of secondary infections. Prophylactic antibiotic therapy is prescribed.

- Debridement or removal of necrotic tissue with skin grafting facilitates healing.

- Early administration of total parenteral nutrition minimizes caloric and nutrient deficits with major burns.

Unit 5

Care of Individuals with High Acuity Neurological Conditions

T*his unit addresses a variety of high acuity neurological and intracranial conditions associated with varying degrees of impaired neurological function. This information follows the previous unit on circulatory/perfusion because an interrelationship exists between cardiac function and the adequacy of other body systems. When the heart can no longer pump sufficient quantities of oxygenated blood into general circulation, the brain is the first organ to experience dysfunction. In turn, neurological dysfunction affects the optimal function of other body systems.*

Persons with high acuity neurological and intracranial conditions were traditionally treated for long periods of time in critical care units. As the trends in health care delivery shift to alternative care settings, persons with high acuity neurological conditions will be transferred earlier in their convalescence to skilled nursing facilities, rehabilitation centers and home health care.

An understanding of general medical-surgical nursing care of neurological conditions provides the basis for the information presented in this unit. The pre-requisite understanding includes normal anatomical and physiological considerations of the central and peripheral nervous system, dynamics of increased intracranial pressure (IICP), and the elements of a neurological assessment. The extension, elaboration and refinement of these concepts provide the foundation for nursing care of high acuity neurological conditions.

Section 1: REVIEW AND OVERVIEW

The neurological system coordinates the internal physiological functioning of other body systems and determines the ability of the body to respond to its surroundings. The central nervous system (CNS) includes the brain and spinal cord. The peripheral nervous system (PNS) includes the cranial and spinal nerves which interact with the musculoskeletal system for sensory input and body movement.

Anatomical and Physiological Review

The rigid, bony compartments of the skull and vertebral column protect the components of the central and peripheral nervous systems. The fibrous coverings (meninges) and cerebrospinal fluid also provide cushioning protection.

1. The cerebrospinal fluid (CSF) circulates around the brain and spinal cord in a space between two meninges—the arachnoid mater and pia mater. Approximately 600-800 ml of CSF forms daily from tiny vessels in the lateral ventricles of the cerebrum. The average amount of CSF in circulation at any time is 130 ml. CSF flows through the subarachnoid space and reabsorbs back into the venous system through the choroid villi on the surface of the brain.

   • Brain volume, blood, and cerebrospinal fluid determine intracranial pressure. Changes in blood vessel size and CSF production accommodate increases/decreases in brain volume to maintain the desired balance. A sudden increase of 5-6 ml or greater in any of these components increases intracranial pressure and impairs cellular function.

2. The cerebrum — the largest portion of the CNS — consists of lobes and hemispheres. The surface, or cortex, has an irregular appearance with raised convolutions (gyri) and recessed furrows (sulci).

- The external surface of the brain and spinal cord consists of gray matter which includes nerve cell bodies and some axons. The white matter or myelinated nerve endings (dendrites and axons) comprises the internal segments of the brain and spinal cord. Myelinated neural tissue has the capability of regeneration following injury.

- Hemispheres connect with a fibrous band of white matter called the corpus callosum. Neural pathways between the hemispheres and the peripheral nervous system ensure coordinated sensory and motor function.

3. Cranial nerves exit the brain through openings in the skull. Each nerve has a specific function, and changes in pressure and volume within the skull affect those functions. Clinical manifestations reflect dysfunction specific to each cranial nerve. Assessment data is valuable for the identification of specific intracranial pathology.

   - Alteration in cranial nerve function produces responses on the side of the body where the nerve is located. For example, pressure on the right third cranial nerve produces sluggish pupillary response in the right eye (ipsilateral response).

4. Peripheral nerve pathways cross from the origin in the brain to the opposite side producing sensory and/or motor responses on the opposite side of the body (contralateral response). For example, a hematoma on the left motor pathway of the frontal lobe produces right hemiparesis.

   - Upper motor neurons (pyramidal cells) have their cell bodies in the motor cortex of the brain. Their axons form pathways along the spinal cord and connect with the peripheral nervous system. On the other hand, the location of the cell bodies of lower motor neurons occurs in the spinal cord or brain stem.

— Coordinated skeletal muscular activity requires the interaction between upper and lower motor neurons. Voluntary muscle response is lost with lower motor neuron dysfunction.

5. Spinal nerves emerge from the spinal cord between each vertebrae. Spinal nerves have both sensory (afferent) and motor (efferent) fibers. Each nerve synapses with specific peripheral nerves and selected skeletal muscles which accompany specific functions. (Refer to the dermatome chart for spinal nerve related function.)

   • Stimulation and response of peripheral nerves may travel to and from the spinal cord producing an involuntary activity (spinal arc reflex). The impulses may also travel along ascending and descending spinal pathways connecting the peripheral nervous system with the brain. Perception and interruption of these impulses permit voluntary activity.

6. The brain requires a constant supply of glucose and oxygen for optimal metabolic activity. Because the brain has minimal storage capacity for both oxygen and glucose, 20% of cardiac output from each heartbeat goes to the brain. Any disruption of cardiac effectiveness or cerebral circulation may lead to cerebral ischemia, hypoxia, and cell damage.

7. **Age Variations:**

   • Variations related to the elderly:

     — In the elderly, reaction time and the time it takes to learn are prolonged and the threshold for activation of sensory receptors is higher.

     — Visual and/or hearing impairment among some elderly contribute to inappropriate responses and may be misinterpreted as confusion or disorientation.

     — A minor fall may cause injury to brain tissue from decreased brain fluid volume and increased adherence of the meninges to the skull. An impact/rebound injury tears tiny vessels on the surface of the brain.

— Restriction of chest movement and ventilatory capacity may occur because of degenerated intervertebral discs and osteoporosis of vertebral bodies.

— Changes in hypothalamus functioning may lead to age-related alterations in sleep/wakefulness and regulation of body temperature. Most elders sleep frequently for short periods. As their normal body temperature is typically below the accepted normal limits, it rises more slowly in response to infection and peaks with lower values. Thus, an elevated temperature of 100° F. is often regarded as not being important when, in fact, a serious infection may be present.

• Variations related to infants and children:

— In these younger age groups, subtle signs of increased intracranial pressure (IICP) often appear before the classic signs seen in adults. Gradual increases in intracranial volume produce bulging fontanelles and separation of cranial sutures or increased head circumference in infants.

— Other subtle signs include lethargy, decreased eye contact with care provider, and changes in feeding behavior. Unilateral ptosis often accompanies ipsilateral pupillary dilation.

— Infants and children can slip into a coma undetected because their normal sleeping pattern includes frequent napping and long sleeping periods. Therefore, assessment following a head injury requires interruption of sleep.

— Blood loss which affects the MAP and, in turn, optimal cerebral perfusion, is commonly underestimated.

— Rhythmic or repetitive nonpurposeful movements of the limbs may represent seizure activity and warrant further evaluation.

— Children with acute increased intracranial pressure (IICP) may develop neurogenic pulmonary edema. Symptoms of congested lung sounds and decreased left heart function may develop suddenly. Early recognition of this complication and restoration of circulatory perfusion maintains desirable cerebral perfusion.

Section 2: PATHOPHYSIOLOGICAL DYSFUNCTION

Etiological factors which contribute to intracranial dysfunction include direct injury to brain tissue, cardiopulmonary dysfunction, tumor growth, intracranial infection, and fever. These factors contribute to increased intracranial pressure (IICP) via different routes. In spite of the etiological factors, IICP interferes with the supply of oxygen, glucose, and nutrients to ensure optimal neural cellular metabolism. Because virtually no storage or reserves of nutrients are within neural tissue, a disruption of supply quickly results in irreversible cellular damage.

1. When a head injury occurs, tissue is damaged beneath the point of impact. Inflammatory response with localized edema takes place around the injured tissue. The injured and inflamed tissue compresses the blood vessels in the area.

   • As the blood supply distal to this injured site diminishes, tissue ischemia and hypoxia results. Cerebral capillary permeability increases and intravascular fluid moves from the capillaries into the interstitial space. Generalized cerebral edema develops and raises IICP.

     — Interstitial edema compresses additional blood vessels and widens the area of cerebral edema. The cycle of damaged tissue leading to additional tissue damage continues unless interventions are successful.

2. When cardiopulmonary dysfunction occurs, decreased pumping effectiveness of the myocardium leads to decreased cardiac output. In turn, the arterial blood supply to the brain decreases.

- As the supply of oxygenated blood to the brain decreases, cerebral tissue ischemia and hypoxia develop. Capillary permeability increases which leads to fluid shifts from the intravascular space to the cerebral interstitial space. Cerebral edema develops.

- Decreased cerebral blood supply slows cerebral circulation. Carbon dioxide, formed from cellular metabolism, accumulates in the blood. Cerebral vasodilation occurs in response to elevated carbon dioxide levels within cerebral circulation. Intravascular blood volume and intracranial volume increase. This sequence of events contributes to increased intracranial pressure.

3. When an intracranial infection occurs, neural cellular metabolism increases. The requirements for oxygen and glucose also increase. If cellular needs exceed the ability to deliver these nutrients, a metabolic deficit occurs. A state of altered cellular metabolism and tissue hypoxia develops.

- The infectious process causes the release of endotoxins which produces a state of generalized vasodilation. Increased capillary permeability leads to a fluid shift from the intravascular space to the interstitial space. The resultant cerebral edema leads to IICP.

4. Primary and metastatic brain tumors increase intracranial volume. Pressure on surrounding tissue initially interferes with electrical impulse transmission leading to seizure activity. Compression of neural tissue alters physiological function and impairs cerebral circulation. IICP expands.

Patho-Development of IICP

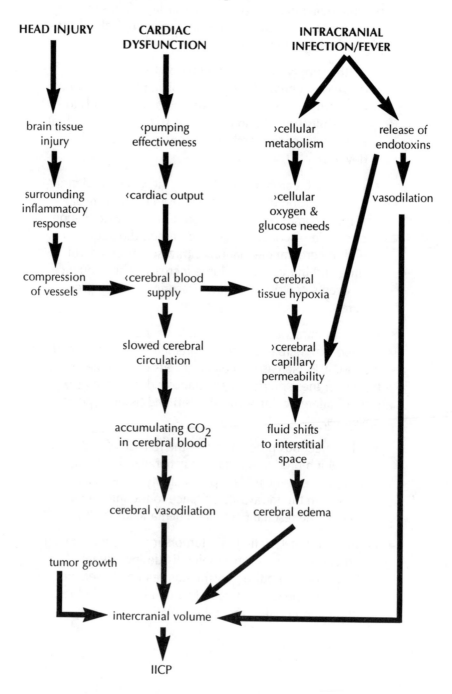

Section 3: DIAGNOSTIC TECHNIQUES AND INTERVENTIONS

Guidelines for Neurological Assessment

The bedside nurse is pivotal in detecting early and subtle changes in neurological status. Accurate assessment and prompt reporting of findings are essential to the appropriate intervention and a favorable outcome. The severity and acuity of neurological status determine the frequency of assessment. An acute and potentially serious intracranial condition warrants frequent assessment (every 10-15 minutes) to detect early changes and subtle trends in status. As a condition stabilizes, the interval between assessments should be lengthened to permit periods of undisturbed rest and eliminate unnecessary neurological stimulation.

Clinical manifestations suggesting an onset of neurological dysfunction warranting further assessment include:

- Restlessness with increasing difficulty concentrating on current activities

- Increasing difficulty waking up or staying awake

- Numbness or weakness on one side of the face or body

- Unexplained seizure or involuntary muscular twitching

Patho Effects of IICP

Anatomy Involved	Clinical Manifestations
Cerebrum	Decreased LOC; headache; seizures
Frontal Lobes • Prefrontal Area • Precentral Gyrus	Personality changes • Alteration in purposeful behavior • Skeletal muscle weakness/paralysis

Anatomy Involved	Clinical Manifestations
Temporal Lobes • Wernecke's Area • Broca's Area	Memory loss • Receptive aphasia • Motor aphasia
Parietal Lobes	Distorted sensory responses
Occipital Lobes	Visual disturbances
3rd Cranial Nerve	Sluggish pupillary response
Hypothalamus	Poor temperature regulation; wide pulse pressure (BP changes); bradycardia
Pons and Brain Stem	Decorticate posturing
Medulla	Respiratory irregularity
Cerebellum	Ataxia; poor coordination
Posterior Pituitary Gland	Profound diuresis of dilute urine
Aqueduct of Sylvius or Pons	Obstructed CSF flow and dilated ventricles

1. Glasgow Coma Scale (GCS):

- The assessment of acute neurological dysfunction and depth of coma follows a widely used standardized guide (GCS). A person's BEST response for eye movements, verbal response and motor function receives a designated numerical value. A total score is valuable in determining the severity of neurological damage and possible prognosis. High total scores accompany good outcome and prognosis; conversely, a low score of 7 typically accompanies severe brain damage and a poor prognosis.

- BEST Verbal Response. When asked, "What day or year is this?" the person responds with:

  — Correct statement of the day of the week or year = "oriented" or 5 points.

  — Incorrect statement of the day of the week or year = "confused" or 4 points.

  — Verbal response which is not related to the question asked = "inappropriate" or 3 points.

  — Moaning or mumbling in response to tactile stimulus = "incomprehensible" or 2 points.

  — No audible response to painful stimulus = "none" or 1 point.

- BEST Eye-Opening Response — When speaking to this person, the response is:

  — Opens eyes and looks at the speaker when spoken to = "spontaneous" or 4 points.

  — Slowly opens eyes after being asked to do so = "to speech" or 3 points.

  — Opens eyes only following painful stimulus = "to pain" or 2 points.

  — No eye opening response = "none" or 1 point.

- BEST Motor Response—When asked to hold up 2 fingers, the response is:

  — Holds up the requested number of fingers with either hand = "obeys" or 6 points.

  — Reaches toward the source or location of the painful stimulus = "localizes" or 5 points.

  — Moves away from the source or location of the painful stimulus = "withdraws" or 4 points.

  — Decorticate posturing to tactile or painful stimulus = "abnormal flexion" or 3 points.

  — Decerebrate posturing to tactile or painful stimulus = "abnormal extension" or 2 points.

  — No response with flaccid muscle tone = "none" or 1 point.

2. **Level of Consciousness (LOC):**

- Assessing a person's ability to understand and respond appropriately follows a sequence of progressive stimulation. Normally, a person responds spontaneously and appropriately to verbal directions. As LOC decreases, response requires increasing verbal and tactile stimulation.

- When no response to verbal stimulation occurs, assessing the response to pain is the next step.

  — Pinching or pricking soft tissue is avoided as bruising may occur.

  — Nailbed pressure with a hard object usually elicits localization or withdrawal from the source of pain. Vigorous rubbing on the sternum usually elicits eye opening or moaning in a comatose patient.

- Assessing for the presence of protective reflex activity is appropriate only when there is a minimal response to painful stimulation. Spontaneous eye blinking indicates the presence of the blink and corneal reflex. Lightly stroking the eyelashes produces reflex blinking activity in most comatose patients. Touching the cornea with a sterile wisp of cotton to assess corneal reflex unnecessarily increases the potential for corneal damage.

- If a person is able to speak, the gag reflex is present. Touching the posterior oropharyngeal fossa or the posterior tongue may produce vomiting and unnecessary increases in intracranial pressure (ICP).

3. **Pupillary responses:**

- Pupils normally constrict to a light stimulus which indicates the normal functioning of cranial nerve III. PERRLA refers to "pupils equal, round, reactive to light accommodation."

- When IICP produces sufficient pressure on cranial nerve III, the pupil on the side with the intracranial lesion (ipsilateral) constricts progressively more slowly.

  — Impact/rebound head injury may produce a contrecoup effect. With impact injury, brain tissue may be damaged on the side of impact producing ipsilateral, sluggish pupillary response. Rebound effect may also produce tissue damage on the opposite side of the brain or a contralateral sluggish pupillary response.

- The onset of sluggish pupillary response warrants prompt reporting so that the timely initiation of intervention will minimize the further development of IICP. Note: Pupillary response is generally a late sign of IICP unless a lesion is developing rapidly or there is direct injury to CN III.

- Fixed, dilated (unresponsive) pupils accompany severe pressure and possibly irreversible brain damage.

- Blindness, glaucoma, cataracts, and optical prostheses may interfere with the accuracy of pupillary response as an indicator of IICP.

4. Changes in vital signs:

- Blood pressure trends typically follow a predictable pattern as IICP progresses. In early stages, the systolic pressure elevates and the diastolic pressure decreases causing a widening pulse pressure.

  — With advanced IICP, the systolic pressure falls to shock-like parameters. As the mean systemic arterial pressure (MSAP) falls and ICP increases, cerebral perfusion pressure (CPP) falls. Altered cerebral cellular metabolism occurs and irreversible brain damage may result.

- Initially, the pulse rate decreases to age-appropriate bradycardia. The character remains full and regular.

  — As IICP progresses, the pulse rate increases to tachycardiac parameters and also becomes weaker. Exacerbation of pre-existing cardiac dysfunction further impairs cerebral perfusion. For example, myocardial ischemia and ectopic beats impair cardiac output and, subsequently, affect cerebral perfusion.

- Infratentorial lesions located in the midbrain, pons, and medulla typically produce alterations in respiratory activity during early stages of IICP.

  — Supratentorial lesions or generalized cerebral edema do not characteristically produce altered breathing patterns until increased intracranial pressure is advanced.

- Difficulty maintaining normal body temperature in the absence of infection is a symptom of pressure on the hypothalamus.

5. Altered motor function:

- Assessing motor response typically accompanies the assessment of LOC. For example, to assess both muscle strength and the person's ability to correctly follow directions (LOC) the nurse may request that the client push his or her feet against the nurse's hand or that the client squeeze the nurse's two fingers.

  — Peripheral motor pathways originating along the precentral gyrus on one hemisphere cross and eventually connect with neuromuscular cells on the opposite side of the body (contralateral response). For example, a lesion or brain injury on the left side of the brain causes right hemiparesis.

- In a person with deep coma and severe brain damage, abnormal motor response (posturing) occurs. Posturing is a generalized involuntary and abnormal response to minimal verbal or tactile stimulation. The characteristic manifestations include rigid extension of the legs and pronation of the feet with rigid flexion or extension of the arms and hands.

  — Decorticate posturing includes spastic flexion of the arms, wrists, and hands toward the midline of the body. The lower extremities maintain rigid extension.

  — Decerebrate posturing includes spastic extension of all extremities and typically accompanies a poor prognosis.

Interventions to control intracranial pressure

1. Airway and gas exchange:

- Ensuring a patent airway is a primary intervention for persons with altered level of consciousness. Since neural tissue is very sensitive to oxygen deficits, achieving an adequate gas exchange is essential to the preservation of cellular functioning.

Decision Tree for Drowsiness
and/or Confusion Following Neurological
Episode

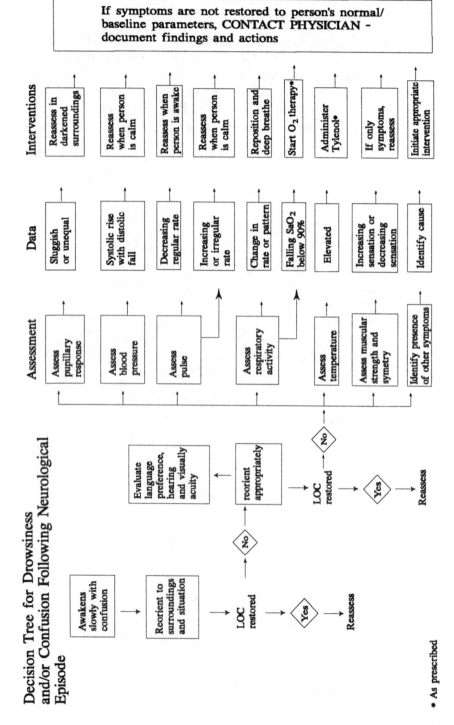

If symptoms are not restored to person's normal/
baseline parameters, CONTACT PHYSICIAN -
document findings and actions

Assessment

Assess pupillary response

Assess blood pressure

Assess pulse

Assess respiratory activity

Assess temperature

Assess muscular strength and symetry

Identify presence of other symptoms

Data

Sluggish or unequal

Systolic rise with distolic fall

Decreasing regular rate

Increasing or irregular rate

Change in rate or pattern

Falling SaO₂ below 90%

Elevated

Increasing sensation or decreasing sensation

Identify cause

Interventions

Reassess in darkened surroundings

Reassess when person is calm

Reassess when person is awake

Reassess when person is calm

Reposition and deep breathe

Start O₂ therapy*

Administer Tylenol*

If only symptoms, reassess

Initiate appropriate intervention

Awakens slowly with confusion

Reorient to surroundings and situation

LOC restored → Yes → Reassess

No

reorient appropriately

Evaluate language preference, hearing and visually acuity

LOC restored → Yes → Reassess

No

* As prescribed

— Coughing and suctioning increase intracranial pressure and may deplete oxygen supply to the brain. Providing 100% FiO_2 prior to suctioning and limiting suctioning to 10-15 seconds minimize the risk of cerebral hypoxia.

• Maintaining therapeutic ABG values often requires mechanical ventilation. A state of hyperventilation is desirable because an elevated $paCO_2$ is a potent cerebral vasodilator. With elevated $paCO_2$ levels, there is an increase in cerebral blood flow and total blood volume within the skull. Increasing the respiratory rate and/or the tidal volume produces hyperventilation. The $paCO_2$ level falls below 35 mmHg and cerebral vessels constrict. As the volume of cerebral blood flow decreases, the intracranial pressure also decreases.

— Desired $paCO_2$ values for acute increased intracranial pressure are: 25-30 mmHg; whereas, normal parameters are 35-45 mmHg.

— Desired paO_2 values are: 80 mmHg to prevent cerebral tissue hypoxia.

2. Intracranial pressure monitoring:

• Establishing a baseline of the clinical manifestations of intracranial pressure is essential and basic to the early recognition of changes. Small increases in volume within the closed compartment of the skull increase the pressure on brain tissue. Fluid, blood, tissue growth, or foreign objects account for an increase in volume.

• Monitoring intracranial pressure provides more precise data on cerebral perfusion pressure (CPP) than the assessment of clinical manifestations. Cerebral perfusion pressure (CPP) equals mean systemic arterial pressure (MSAP) minus intracranial pressure (ICP) or CPP = MSAP- ICP. Within this equation, factors and interventions that raise or decrease ICP have the greatest impact on ensuring optimal cerebral perfusion.

— Optimal cerebral perfusion pressure is: 60-80 mmHg. CPP < 30 mmHg is incompatible with life.

— IICP monitoring is an invasive technique. The tip of a catheter is inserted through a surgical opening in the skull and forwarded to a lateral ventricle, subarachnoid space, or epidural space. The attached pressurized fluid and transducer system is similar to the system used for hemodynamic monitoring. Waveforms and digital readouts on a monitor represent pressures detected at the tip of the catheter.

— If acute, severe pressure occurs and the CPP falls to a critical level, the removal of some cerebrospinal (CSF) is possible via the intraventricular device.

3. Proper head positioning:

• Elevating the head of the bed at 15-30° facilitates cerebral venous drainage. Higher elevations may precipitate downward pressure of intracranial tissue through the openings in the tentorium or foramen (herniation).

• Maintaining the head and neck in an anatomically neutral position with no flexion facilitates optimal arterial and venous circulation. The preferred body position during acute increased intracranial pressure is flat in bed. The use of a pillow under the head increases the risk of neck flexion.

• Maintaining neutral neck alignment with support of the head is essential when turning an individual to either side.

4. Blood pressure control:

• Controlling episodes of hypertension and hypotension decrease the risk of intracranial pressure and cerebral edema. Hypotension decreases the oxygen delivery to brain tissue causing the SaO_2 and pH to fall. Neural tissue ischemia increases capillary permeability which leads to fluid shifts and cerebral interstitial edema. Hypertension and/or wide fluctuations in blood pressure may precipitate cerebral capillary bleeding.

— Arterial and hemodynamic monitoring provide continual data. Fluid therapy, vasopressors, or vasodilators provide pharmacological control of the blood pressure within an acceptable range.

5. **Fluid, nutrient, and electrolyte therapy:**

   • Providing fluid balance with D_5 with saline minimizes cerebral edema which may occur with the administration of D_5W alone. The daily fluid requirements are typically 2/3 of a person's daily maintenance needs. A slightly dehydrated state is desirable. Desired CVP values during acute IICP are within the low normal range (0-3 mmHg). Indirectly, these values minimize the potential for excess fluid volume within the cerebral circulation.

   — An individual's body weight (BW) in kilograms (Kg) determines daily fluid needs. Typically for an adult, an estimate of the total fluid requirements is: the first 10 Kg of BW requires 100 ml per Kg (or 1000 ml); the second 10 Kg of BW requires 50 ml per Kg (or 500 ml); the remaining Kg of BW requires 20 ml per Kg. The recommended daily fluid needs during the acute increased intracranial pressure phase are 2/3 of this total estimated volume.

   • IV administration of potassium supplements meets daily requirements. The administration of other electrolytes is in response to lab findings.

   • Hyperalimentation and intralipids provide caloric needs during the acute phase. Until bowel sounds return, the removal of gastric secretions is essential to minimize the risk of vomiting and aspiration. Enteral feedings are appropriate for individuals with limited LOC and a stabilized intracranial condition.

— The brain virtually has no glucose stores and injured neural cells have higher glucose requirements than noninjured cells. Therefore, hyperalimentation provides these additional energy requirements and minimizes the risk of altered cellular metabolism and the use of tissue protein for energy. Depleted protein stores lead to a state of catabolism and negative nitrogen balance. Delayed tissue healing results.

6. Normothermia:

• Maintaining a normal body temperature ensures optimal cerebral cellular metabolism. An elevated body temperature increases cellular metabolism and the need for oxygen and glucose. The physiological response to a temperature elevation is vasodilation, an increased blood flow and increased cellular metabolism. In a situation of compromised cerebral function, this normal response may increase intracranial volume and, indirectly, increase cerebral edema.

— The administration of antipyretics typically maintains a body temperature within normal range. When a temperature is difficult to control, cooling blankets are beneficial.

— The presence of infection warrants the administration of antibiotics to control the infectious process and secondary inflammatory response.

— The blood-brain barrier which protects the brain from potentially harmful substances inhibits the effectiveness of most antibiotics. Only a few antibiotics penetrate the barrier — penicillin, ampicillin, chloramphenicol and nafcillin. Typically, relatively high IV doses are required to achieve therapeutic effects during an acute neurological infection.

— Shivering associated with an elevated temperature also increases cellular metabolism and requires pharmacological control. Some tranquilizers, such as chlorpromazine, are beneficial.

- A barbiturate coma may minimize cerebral metabolism. When intracranial hypertension is uncontrolled, continued administration of pentobarbital reduces the cerebral metabolic rate. Because of the concurrent depressant effects of this medication, individuals require intubation and mechanical ventilation, arterial line, hemodynamic and intracranial monitoring. The goals include maintaining the systolic BP > 80 mmHg and the CPP between 60-80 mmHg.

7. **Seizure control:**

   - Administering anticonvulsants prophylactically minimizes the risk for seizures, especially when a supratentorial lesion exists.

   - Observation and accurate documentation of seizure activity help to determine the location of intracranial pathology. The pattern of skeletal muscle activity is either localized (tremor or twitch) or vigorous, generalized (grand mal).

     — If consciousness is lost, airway obstruction may develop due to tongue displacement or aspiration of secretions. Cerebral hypoxia may develop with disrupted breathing patterns. Placing an oral airway maintains a patent airway.

     — Intermittent contractions of the jaw muscles may injure the tongue. Placing an oral airway or padded tongue blades between the teeth minimizes injury to the soft tissue of the mouth and tongue.

     — Status epilepticus refers to prolonged and/or continuous seizure activity. This becomes a medical emergency as ICP increases and cerebral hypoxia occurs.

8. **Pharmacological therapy:**

   - Sedatives (phenobarbital) reduce restlessness and irritability which may contribute to elevated blood pressure and increased intracranial pressure.

- Antipyretics control fever and cellular metabolism. Aspirin is avoided because of its propensity for altering the clotting cascade and increasing the risk for bleeding.

- Analgesics relieve pain. Acetaminophen is the preferred medication as it has minimal neurological side effects. Morphine obscures pupillary response and meperidine often precipitates hypotension.

- Corticosteroids (Decadron) is a medication commonly prescribed for its anti-inflammatory and capillary wall stabilizing properties. The literature reports disagreement on its effectiveness. Cautious administration includes close observation for side effects, especially GI irritation and bleeding.

- Osmotic diuretics (mannitol, urea, glycerol) reduce intracranial pressure by producing fluid shifts from the interstitial space into the intravascular compartment. Diuresis and slight hypovolemia result. Continued use often reverses desired fluid shifts and cerebral edema increases rather than decreases.

- Stool softeners minimize straining during defecation (Valsalva response) which may aggravate intracranial pressure.

9. **Care during unconsciousness:**

- During the acute IICP phase, a delicate balance exists among minimal physical stimulation, assessment of neurological status, undisturbed rest, and physical care. With altered LOC, it is often difficult to determine the extent of a person's awareness or passive interaction with the surroundings.

- Hearing is a strong sense that remains intact even when a person is unconscious and displays no obvious physical response. A client with sufficient cerebral electrical impulse transmission has the potential to hear. Persons should be treated as if they can hear until EEG or cerebral angiography verifies that no cerebral activity is present.

— Bedside conversations should include the person as if hearing is intact. Address the person with respect and avoid informal names. Discussions about poor prognosis, other patients, or personal topics are best conducted beyond the person's hearing range.

- Audio tapes of soothing music played intermittently by cassette player and earphone may block environmental noise and promote restful sleep. Audio tapes of encouraging family conversations are equally soothing to some persons.

10. Identification of complications:

- Diabetes insipidus may develop secondarily due to pressure on the posterior pituitary gland. An inadequate release of antidiuretic hormone results in decreased water reabsorption in the kidneys. The excretion of large quantities of free water occurs and profound diuresis of extremely dilute urine results. Severe extracellular and intracellular dehydration, hypotension, and hypovolemic shock develop. The onset is typically sudden and abrupt.

  — If untreated, the excretion of as much as 5-40 liters of urine in a day may occur. Indications include a sudden increase in urinary output of 200 ml/hour despite unchanged fluid intake.

  — Urinary specific gravity is less than 1.007 with increased serum osmolality 300 mOsm/Kg.

  — An associated increase in serum sodium occurs with values 147 mEq/L.

- Treatment includes the administration of vasopressin (exogenous ADH). As side effects include hypertension, there is a delicate balance between dosage and response. Rapid IV fluid replacement restores hemodynamic status.

Section 4: EXAMPLES OF COMMON CLINICAL CONDITIONS

Subarachnoid Hemorrhage

This cerebral hemorrhage results from a bleeding or the rupture of a cerebral aneurysm. An aneurysm is a localized dilation or bulging in the wall of an artery. A cerebral aneurysm is either saccular, a congenital berry-like defect on the side of the artery, or generalized, fusiform bulging associated with atherosclerosis.

- Berry aneurysms typically occur in one component of the Circle of Willis at the base on the brain. This type of aneurysm usually is asymptomatic until early adulthood when an episode of hypertension causes it to bleed. A subarachnoid hemorrhage results from bleeding in the subarachnoid space.

- The fusiform or dissecting cerebral aneurysm results from atherosclerotic involvement of arterioles on the brain surface. This type of cerebral aneurysm occurs in later adult life. Essential hypertension and an acute hypertensive episode precipitates a bleed. An intercerebral hematoma results from bleeding into surrounding brain tissue.

1. Pathophysiology:

- Initially after the bleed, the vessel temporarily vasoconstricts resulting in decreased cerebral blood flow. The subsequent distal ischemia contributes to neurologic deficit. The degree of vasospasm correlates to the degree of cerebral bleed.

  — Vasospasm typically peaks 7-10 days following the initial bleed and, if uncomplicated, resolves in approximately 3 weeks. Some cerebral bleeds

result in irreversible brain damage. Surgical ligation corrects some bleeding sites.

— When the vasospasm relaxes, the vessel may
rebleed. The risk for this complication is greatest
24-48 hours following the initial bleed.
Rebleeding may occur as late as 6 months later.

— Thrombosis formation occurs in the constricted
vessel resulting in permanently impaired circulation distal to the affected segment (cerebral infarction). Lysis or dissolving of the thrombosis
normally occurs 7-10 days after the original bleed
and vasospasm. The risk of rebleed is also
increased during this 7-10 day time period.

— Collateral circulation around the vasospasm and
thrombosed site gradually provides a secondary
blood supply around the affected area. This physiological mechanism permits the resolution of secondary inflammatory edema but cannot restore
irreversible neurological damage.

• If the initial bleed and subsequent impaired cerebral
perfusion is extensive, irreversible damaged brain tissue and severe neurological impairment occurs.
Brain death is another possibility. (Refer to Unit 1:
"Concepts Common to High Acuity Nursing Care"
for additional information on brain death.)

2. **Indications:**

• Early clinical manifestations include: meningeal irritation due to presence of blood in the subarachnoid
space; nuchal rigidity (stiff neck); headache; photo-
phobia; lethargy; vomiting without nausea.

— Persons describe the headaches as "the worst ever
experienced" and like an "explosion going off in
my head."

— Early signs of increased intracranial pressure:
decreasing LOC; elevated systolic and decreased

diastolic blood pressure; bradycardia; ipsilateral decreased pupillary response.

- International grading system (1-5) permits objective and comparative evaluation of symptoms. Grades 4 and 5 have high morbidity and mortality outcomes.

3. Medical and Nursing Management:

- Surgical ligation of the aneurysm or affected vessel is possible for stabilized clinical situations with low staging (1-3).

- Interventions focus on minimizing intracranial pressure through methods such as complete bedrest with restricted activities, neutral head position, 15-30 degree HOB elevation, intracranial pressure neurological assessment, and pharmacological management.

  — The use of antifibrinolytic agents (Amicar) prevents physiological lysis of the thrombosis at the aneurysm site. The delay of spontaneous breakdown of the thrombosis provides time for further physiological stabilization and preparation for surgical ligation.

Antihypertensive agents reduce the blood pressure and the risk of rebleeding. Commonly prescribed medications include hydralazine hydrochloride (Apresoline), methyldopa (Aldomet), or reserpine.

Head Injury

Impact accidents are the primary cause of head injuries with the highest incidence occurring in young adult males. The extent of damage at the time of impact and the time interval between injury and the initiation of treatment determine the outcome. Long-term disability is profound. Each survivor of a severe head injury requires between $4.1 million and $9 million in care over a lifetime. National Institutes of Health estimates that 70,000-90,000 survivors per year remain in coma or suffer extreme loss of body functions.

Primary injury relates directly to the impact and the resulting damage. This injury includes concussion (edema), contusion (bruising), laceration, and/or skull fracture. Secondary intracranial injury follows the primary injury and includes hematoma formation, intracranial hypertension, CNS infection, and/or cerebral edema. Secondary extracranial injury results from systemic hypotension, hypoxia, and/or hypercapnia. The presence of secondary events accounts for poorer recovery and higher risk of mortality.

1. **Pathophysiology:**

   - As with tissue injury elsewhere in the body, the inflammatory response produces varying degrees of interstitial edema surrounding the injured site. When this response occurs within the closed compartment of the skull, only small increases (5 ml) in intracranial volume result in profound pressure increases.

     — Pressure increases impair perfusion to neural tissue and alter cellular metabolism. As neural glucose and oxygen stores are minimal, impaired metabolism rapidly progresses to irreversible brain damage.

   - Lesions that occur above the tentorium (supratentorial) may interfere with the electrical impulse transmission along cerebral pathways thereby increasing the risk for seizures.

   - Lesions that occur below the tentorium (infratentorial) may interfere with impulse transmission between the cerebrum and the rest of the body. The risk for dysfunction of the vital centers located in the medulla also increases.

   - Injury to blood vessels on the surface of the brain may produce a hematoma either above or below the dura mater (meninges). An epidural hematoma occurs above the dura mater from an arteriolar bleed. These hematomas usually develop rapidly. A subdural hematoma occurs below the dura mater from a slow venous bleed.

• Herniation of intracranial structures may accompany a sudden increase in intracranial pressure. Secondary edema or localized bleeding is typically the underlying cause of herniation. Astute nursing assessment for the early signs of herniation and facilitating prompt intervention are essential in preventing irreversible damage.

— Uncal herniation occurs when an expanding supratentorial lesion in the region of the temporal lobe produces pressure over the tentorium and adjacent midbrain. The expanding lesion compresses the third cranial nerve and posterior cerebral artery on the same side as the expanding pressure.

— Central or transtentorial herniation occurs when the hemisphere protrudes through the tentorial notch. Compression of the midbrain, pons, and medulla produces life-threatening changes in physiological function. Clinical signs are respirations which progress to Cheyne-Stokes pattern. Pupils initially may be small and reactive to light and later become unequal or misshapen and progress to fixed and dilated.

Focused Bedside Assessment

The following guideline provides data expected from a head-to-toe assessment of an individual experiencing IICP. This example focuses on a supratentorial head injury. Pathophysiological problems involving other body systems are not included.

- **General Appearance:** sleeping when not aroused; at risk for seizures; headache.

- **Level of Consciousness:** easily aroused from sleeping state; oriented to person, place but not time. *Progressive signs:* more stimulation required to arouse; decreasing orientation (confusion or disorientation); withdraws or localizes to painful stimulation. *Serious signs:* Only moans to painful stimulation; abnormal posturing.

- **Head and Neck:** pupils constrict equally to light; clear drainage from nose or ears that tests positive for glucose is CSF; may exhibit bruising/ecchymosis of eyelids (raccoon's eyes); may exhibit bruising/ecchymosis of mastoid area (Battle's sign). *Progressive signs:* sluggish pupillary constriction or unequal response; nuchal rigidity. *Serious signs:* unresponsive (fixed) pupillary response; dilated or constricted pupils.

- **Cardiac Status:** rate and rhythm WNL. *Progressive signs:* elevating systolic with decreasing diastolic blood pressure; bradycardia. *Serious signs:* shock-like pattern; falling blood pressure with elevating pulse rate.

- **Respiratory Status:** gas exchange WNL; typically slow, deep regular breathing; yawning associated with decreased cerebral oxygenation. *Progressive signs:* airway obstruction from tongue accompanies decreased LOC and coma; altered gas exchange secondary to degree of altered ventilation. *Serious signs:* altered respiratory pattern; Cheyne-Stoke pattern; apneic episodes.

- **Abdominal Status:** findings WNL; forceful (projectile) vomiting without nausea is possible. *Progressive signs:* decreased peristalsis leading to diminished bowel sounds.

- **Urinary Elimination:** WNL and appropriate to fluid intake. *Serious signs:* progressive diuresis of dilute urine in spite of unchanged fluid intake (diabetes insipidus).

- **Extremities:** appropriately moves extremities to verbal commands. *Progressive signs:* weakness or paralysis associated with location of intracranial injury (ipsilateral or contralateral). *Serious signs:* decerebrate or decorticate posturing.

When the person is turned to his/her side, the nurse assesses no unusual findings. If additional data is observed, a more detailed assessment of the involved system is required. Additional areas of physiological dysfunction may be present and confound the present intracranial and neurological problem.

- Characteristic clinical manifestations of a basilar skull fracture include raccoon's eyes (periorbital ecchymosis), Battle's sign (mastoid ecchymosis), and CSF drainage from the ears or nose.

  — CSF differs from clear drainage from the nose (rhinorrhea). In a dipstick test for glucose, CSF tests positive and rhinorrhea tests negative.

- Characteristic clinical manifestations of an epidural hematoma include brief loss of consciousness followed by orientation, severe vomiting often without nausea, intense headache, and rapidly decreasing LOC.

- Hematoma formation, contusion and concussion occur on the same side as the point of impact (ipsilateral) or on the opposite side (contralateral). Contrecoup refers to an impact and secondary reactive/rebound displacement injury. In this situation, pathology may occur on the side of injury and on the opposite side as result of impact and rebound movement of intracranial structures.

- Characteristic clinical manifestations of a subdural hematoma include progressive disorientation, persistent headache, increasing lethargy, and personality changes.

- Characteristic clinical manifestations of a concussion — a localized bruise of the brain — include transient loss of consciousness, memory loss, dizziness, headache. Recurrent headaches, flashing lights, or transient visual disturbances may persist for several days, weeks, or months following injury.

- Characteristic clinical manifestations of a contusion include loss of consciousness and sensory/motor disturbances related to the site involved. These clinical manifestations resemble those associated with hematoma formation.

3. Medical and Nursing Management:

- The focus of all interventions is to minimize the progression of IICP. The intervention is determined through close monitoring of neurological status. Refer to an earlier section in this unit for discussion of the possible interventions.

Acute Spinal Cord Injury (SCI)

A spinal cord injury results from an impact accident which produces a concussion, contusion, laceration, or hemorrhage within the vertebral column. Approximately 15,000-20,000 new SCI's occur per year resulting in permanent paraplegia or quadriplegia. Although the postinjury life expectancy is good, morbidity and mortality are due to secondary infection. Renal and pulmonary complications account for 30-40% of all postinjury deaths.

1. Pathophysiology:

- SCI's typically are described according to location of the vertebral and spinal nerve involvement. Each pair of spinal nerves exits the vertebral column and connects with specific motor and sensory nerves in the skeletal muscles. The presence or absence of characteristic data validate the site and severity of spinal cord damage.

- Secondary edema surrounding the specific site of cord damage produces more profound symptoms. As the edema subsides, the determination of a complete or incomplete lesion is possible. "Complete" refers to the absence of all voluntary motor, sensory, and vasomotor function below the level of injury. "Incomplete" refers to the presence of some percentage of intact function below the level of injury.

- Spinal shock occurs immediately following injury. Due to complete neurovascular shutdown, all reflex activity below the level of injury is lost or absent. This response may last minutes, days, or weeks. The more quickly signs of returning function appear, the better the prognosis for restored function.

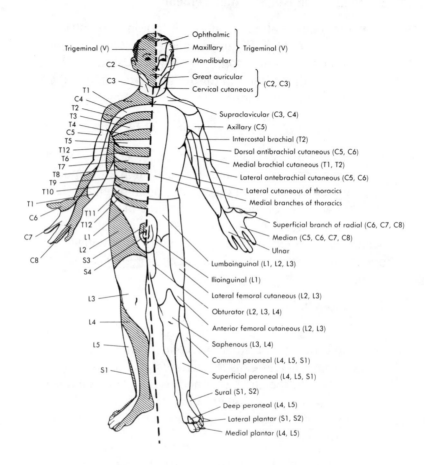

Peripheral distribution of sensory nerve fibers (anterior view). Right, distribution of cutaneous nerves. Left, dermatomes (shaded) or segmental distribution of cutaneous nerves. From W. J. Phipps, B.C. Long, N. F. Woods: Medical-Surgical Nursing: Concepts and Clinical Practices, 3rd Ed; St. Louis: Mosby-Year Book, Inc. 1987. Reprinted with permission

2. Indications:

- Acute signs of spinal shock include the following findings below the level of injury: flaccid paralysis, absence of deep tendon reflexes (DTR), absence of cutaneous sensation, urinary and fecal retention, unstable blood pressure, and absence of sweating.

— Hypotension is due to profound vasodilation in the structures below the level of injury. The higher the level of injury, especially high cervical injury, the greater the peripheral vasodilation and hypotension (normovolemic shock or neurogenic shock).

— Loss of sympathetic response causes venous pooling and decreased blood return to the heart. Flaccid paralysis of skeletal muscles contributes to decreased venous return.

• Characteristic clinical manifestations by levels of cord injury are:

— **C4 and higher:** Loss of all skeletal muscle function, including all muscles for respiration. With a complete cord transection, the individual often expires at the scene of the accident unless immediately ventilated mechanically.

— **C4-5:** Some loss of all skeletal muscle function including the intercostal muscles for respiration. The phrenic nerve is intact and permits spontaneous diaphragmatic breathing. Assisted ventilation is required.

— **C6-8:** Quadriplegia with increased respiratory function. Some movement, but minimal strength of the neck, shoulders, chest, and upper arms is possible. Independent breathing produces normal gas exchange and ventilation, but the cough reflex is often weak or ineffectual for expectorating sputum.

— **T1-3:** Neck, shoulder, chest, arm, hand, and respiratory function is present and more effective. Maintaining a sitting position without support is difficult.

— **T4-10:** More stability of the trunk muscles is possible. The lower the lesion, the greater the independence and improvement in respiratory function. Paraplegia is present.

— **T11-12:** The use of the upper extremities, neck, and shoulders is generally good. Chest and trunk muscles provide stability for upper body movement. Loss of voluntary bowel and bladder control with reflex emptying occurs. Men often experience difficulty attaining and maintaining penile erection. Minimal seminal emission occurs.

— **L3-S1:** All muscle groups in the upper body and most in the lower extremities provide functional use. Loss of voluntary bowel and bladder function with reflex emptying continues. Men often experience diminished penile erection ability with diminished seminal emission.

— **S2-4**: All muscle groups function with some weakness in the lower extremities. Bowel and bladder flaccidity occurs resulting in retention problems. Male impotence may persist.

3. Medical and Nursing Management:

- Initial treatment focuses on stabilization of the injured site. Skeletal traction immobilizes and reduces the fracture or dislocation. For cervical injuries, tongs are attached to the skull. Alignment is achieved through the use of weights attached to ropes and pulleys. Halo devices and fiberglass jackets immobilize the vertebral column.

- A decompression laminectomy relieves pressure or removes bone fragments. Spinal fusion or the insertion of Harrington rods provides vertebral stabilization for high spinal injuries.

- Individuals with cervical injuries require respiratory support. An ineffective cough or difficulty expectorating sputum increase the risk of respiratory infection. Aggressive pulmonary care minimizes this complication.

- Indwelling or intermittent catheterization decompresses a flaccid/atonic bladder during the immediate postinjury phase. When spinal shock resolves, individuals with injury above T12 generally develop a reflex neurogenic bladder which fills and empties automatically. With injuries below T12, individuals develop an areflexic neurogenic bladder which overfills causing overflow incontinence with residual. Intermittent catheterization routine minimizes incontinence and bladder infections.

- Orthostatic hypotension often is a permanent problem, especially for individuals with cervical and high thoracic injuries. Due to ineffective vessel response below the level of injury, intravascular volume shifts follow gravity. Sudden movement to an upright position results in intravascular fluid shifts downward toward the extremities producing a sudden fall in blood pressure. Cerebral hypoxia and loss of consciousness occur. Abdominal binders and thigh-high antiembolic stockings minimize this problem.

- Autonomic dysreflexia (AD) occurs in 80% of individuals with lesions at or above T6. This life-threatening episode is an exaggerated sympathetic nervous system response to a systemic stimulus.

  — The most common causes relate to urinary bladder, bowel, and skin factors. Bladder triggering stimuli include distention, infection, or calculi. Fecal impaction, rectal exam or suppository insertion may trigger the response. Tight clothing, temperature extremes, or areas of broken skin are additional triggering factors.

  — Characteristic symptoms include throbbing headache, cutaneous vasodilation, and profuse sweating above the level of injury. Systemic symptoms include hypertension (typically 250/150 mmHg), blurred vision, nausea, and bradycardia. Symptoms below the level of injury include pilomotor erection ("goose bumps"), pallor, chills, and vasoconstriction.

— Treatment focuses on removing or relieving the causative stimulus. Systemic symptoms usually subside with the elimination of the triggering factor. Sometimes circulatory responses require medication to minimize the adverse effects.

Carotid Insufficiency

Atherosclerotic plaques narrow the opening of the carotid arteries. Carotid insufficiency is a result of this narrowing. Progressive decrease in blood flow to the brain occurs. Episodes of sudden decrease in cerebral blood flow or transient ischemic attacks (TIA) also may occur.

1. Pathophysiology:

- Atherosclerotic plaques invade the vessel wall and progressively weaken it. Underlying or pre-existing hypertension exerts increased pressure on these affected vascular areas.

2. Indications:

- Altered blood flow to the brain produces episodes of altered LOC or transient ischemic attacks (TIA). Fainting accompanied by some transient memory loss and minimal muscle weakness are characteristic clinical manifestations.

- Palpated bruit over the affected area results from the turbulent blood flow over the irregular surface of the affected vessel.

- Angiographic studies identify the location and severity of occlusion.

3. Medical and Nursing Management:

- Carotid endarterectomy refers to the surgical removal of the plaque.

  — During the initial post-operative period, monitoring the systolic blood pressure is essential. Sustained hypertension exerts potentially dangerous pressure on the operative site and weakened vessel wall. An episode of severe hypertension may cause bleeding from the operative site (carotid bleed).

  — The intravenous administration of nitroprusside (Nipride) controls the systolic pressure within pre-operative parameters.

  — Post-op management includes frequent checks of airway. Swelling can lead to stridor and compromised respirations.

- There is a potential risk for plaque fragments to dislodge and travel along the cerebral vascular system. When a fragment lodges in a smaller arteriole, it occludes the vessel like a thrombosis or cerebral vascular accident (CVA).

Infectious Conditions

CNS infections include meningitis (involving the coverings/meninges of the brain or spinal cord), encephalitis (involving brain tissue), or localized infections (abscess formation). These infections also produce inflammatory swelling and increased blood flow within the skull or vertebral column. The degree of increased intracranial pressure corresponds to the severity of the infectious process.

1. Pathophysiology:

- Infective microorganisms may invade the central nervous system from the blood stream, from a penetrating trauma, or by extension of an ear or sinus infection.

— The blood-brain barrier protects brain tissue from potentially harmful substances and microorganism invasion. Therefore, only a few microorganisms can penetrate this barrier from the blood and cause an infection of brain tissue. Meningitis, an infection of the coverings (meninges), is a common neurological infection. Bacterial meningitis is a medical emergency as it has a high mortality rate.

• Swelling of the meninges and the potential scarring may interfere with the reabsorption of CSF. An excess accumulation of CSF within the subarachnoid space and ventricles may occur (acquired hydrocephalus).

2. Indications:

• Common symptoms of bacterial meningitis include: fever, severe headache, nuchal rigidity, increased intracranial pressure, and seizures.

— Examination of the CSF obtained by lumbar puncture confirms the diagnosis. Elevated CSF protein levels and decreased CSF glucose occur. CSF pressure is elevated, and the fluid appears cloudy.

3. Medical and Nursing Management:

• The administration of sufficient quantities of antibiotics to control the infectious process is difficult because the blood-brain barrier minimizes the movement of antibiotics to the infected tissue. Only a few antibiotics penetrate the barrier: penicillin, ampicillin, chloramphenicol, nafcillin.

• During an acute neurological infection, the appropriate antibiotic is administered in relatively high doses, evenly divided over each 24-hour period. The goal is to achieve and maintain high blood levels of the antibiotic. Introduction of an antibiotic into the subarachnoid space (intrathecal route) may be required to achieve the desired outcome.

UNIT 6

Care of Individuals with High Acuity Renal Conditions

This unit addresses various high acuity renal conditions which are typically noted as complications from inadequate perfusion of the kidneys. Persons with altered renal function traditionally were cared for in critical care units or specialized renal dialysis units. However, as the trends of health care delivery shift to ambulatory, extended, and home health settings, the principles of high acuity renal nursing care and related nursing interventions will extend beyond the walls of the traditional acute care hospital.

The information presented in this unit focuses on acute renal failure and the multiple system involvement accompanying chronic renal failure. An understanding of general renal and urinary elimination nursing care is the basis for information in this unit. This prerequisite understanding includes normal anatomical and physiological function of the kidneys and urinary tract as well as the assessment of uncomplicated renal function. An extension, elaboration, and refinement of these fundamental concepts provides the basis of high acuity renal nursing care.

Section 1: REVIEW AND OVERVIEW

The kidneys and urinary tract form an efficient filtering and regulatory system. Adequate renal function is closely interrelated with the functioning of other body systems. For example, cardiac dysfunction, with the associated decreased cardiac output, directly affects the filtrating capacity of the kidneys. In a similar manner, renal dysfunction, with subsequent inadequate fluid or electrolyte elimination, leads to impaired perfusion of nutrients and cellular dysfunction of various organs.

Anatomical Review

The working unit of the kidney is the nephron. Each adult kidney contains approximately 1.2 million nephrons. Each nephron consists of the filtering component (glomerulus) and the tubular network (proximal, Loop of Henle, convoluted and distal tubules). A tiny ball-like structure (Bowman's capsule) encompasses the glomerulus and the renal arterioles.

1. Filtration and regulation of fluid, nutrients, and electrolytes occur within each glomerulus. The wall of the renal afferent arterioles and the epithelial lining of the glomerulus form a semi-permeable membrane. Various physiological factors and pressure differences determine the degree of filtration across this membrane.

2. Blood flows from the glomerulus to the tubular network via efferent arterioles. The vessels surrounding the tubules permit the reabsorption of selected amounts of fluid, nutrients, and electrolytes from the filtrate back into the circulation. Various physiological factors determine the degree of reabsorption.

3. The fluid, nutrients, and electrolytes not reabsorbed from the filtrate flow along the tubules and drain into the urinary tract for elimination as urine.

Physiological Review

The primary purpose of the renal system is to maintain a stable internal environment for optimal cellular and body system activity. A balanced state occurs by regulating fluids, electrolytes, and acid-base, excreting metabolic waste products and erythropoiesis.

1. Fluid regulation:

- The kidneys are very vascular. They receive 1000-1200 ml of blood/minute or 20-25% of each heartbeat (cardiac output). Renal blood flow (RBF) or renal perfusion refers to the amount of blood that passes through each kidney 600 ml/minute. Various physiological factors affect the adequacy of renal blood supply.

- Glomerular filtration rate (GFR) refers to the amount of fluid and substances that pass from the afferent renal arterioles through the semi-permeable membrane into the glomerulus. Filtrate is the fluid and substances that gather in the glomerulus. A normal GFR is 125 ml/minute or 7.5 liters/hour. This filtrate flows from the glomerulus into the tubular network where selective reabsorption occurs.

  — 99% of the filtrate moves from the tubules back into circulation. Only 1%, or a few milliliters, remain in the tubules to form the urine.

  — The normal volume of urine formed and excreted daily for an adult is 1000-2000 ml. Fluid intake and metabolic processes affect the volume of urine. The minimal acceptable amount of urine is 30 ml/hour.

- The renal arterioles constrict and dilate to maintain fairly constant renal blood flow, filtration, and reabsorption rates. This process of autoregulation occurs when the systolic blood pressure is between 80-180 mmHg. Without this protective mechanism, depletion of fluids and electrolytes from the vascular system would occur in less than 5 minutes.

- The sympathetic neural impulses which cause vasoconstriction also influence renal blood flow. For example, when the systemic systolic blood pressure falls below 80 mmHg, the renal arteries constrict and RBF decreases. A subsequent decrease in filtration and an increase in reabsorption occurs to ensure adequate intravascular volume and the maintenance of an adequate blood pressure.

  — Physical exercise, body position, and hypoxia trigger a similar response.

  — Hormonal responses also influence vasoconstriction, filtration, and reabsorption. A decrease in renal blood flow triggers the renin-angiotensin-aldosterone cycle. (Refer to Unit 4: "Care of Individuals with High Acuity Circulatory Conditions" for additional information.)

2. Electrolyte regulation:

- Electrolytes are small molecules that readily pass into the glomerulus and move back into circulation from the tubules. Coordinated balance of filtration and selective reabsorption maintain normal serum electrolyte levels. For example, the reabsorption rate for filtered sodium is 99.5% while for filtered potassium the reabsorption rate is 94%

- Electrolyte levels remain relatively constant despite continuous changes in oral intake, renal filtration, and reabsorption. As storages of electrolytes are virtually nonexistent, daily intake and excretion of excesses maintain the serum levels WNL. Although values may vary according to the laboratory equipment used, normal parameters are:

  — Serum potassium   3.5-5.0 mEq/L

  — Serum sodium   135-145 mEq/L

— Serum calcium	4.5-5.8 mEq/L or
	8.5-10.5 mg/dl
— Serum phosphate	3.0-4.5 mg/dl
— Serum magnesium	1.4-2.5 mEq/L

- Glucose molecules also move freely across the membranes in the glomerulus and tubules. When the serum glucose level is greater than 180 mg/dl, excess glucose remains in the tubules and is excreted in the urine. Urine testing for glucose reveals the degree of glucose excess and serves as an indirect estimate of serum glucose levels.

  — Because glucose molecules also attract water molecules, decreased water reabsorption occurs in the tubules. Increased urine production (polyuria) accompanies elevated urine glucose levels. Without adequate fluid intake, dehydration develops.

3. Acid-base regulation:

- Cellular activity produces acids (carbon dioxide, pyruvic or lactic acids) as end or waste products of metabolism. The respiratory and renal systems achieve a balanced acid-base state by facilitating the elimination of metabolic waste products.

- The kidney's filtration and reabsorption capability regulates the balance between hydrogen molecules (acid) and the bicarbonate molecules (base) to maintain a plasma/serum pH of 7.35-7.45. When the serum is alkalotic (pH 7.45), increased reabsorption of hydrogen occurs in the tubules and excess bicarbonate is excreted in the urine. When the serum is acidotic (pH), increased reabsorption of bicarbonate occurs in the tubules and excess hydrogen is excreted in the urine.

  — An additional mechanism occurs within the kidneys to counteract an acidotic state. Kidneys have the capability of generating bicarbonate molecules from available hydrogen, oxygen, and carbon dioxide.

4. Excretion of metabolic waste products:

- Urea and creatinine are end, or waste, products of protein metabolism. The glomerulus freely filters urea from the blood for urinary excretion. As urea is toxic to body tissues — especially the brain — excretion of excess amounts is essential.

  — The presence of urea in the renal filtrate has a secondary positive effect. It contributes to the kidney's ability to concentrate urine by increasing fluid reabsorption. Therefore, individuals with catabolic, protein depleted, or cachectic states are at risk for inadequate urine concentration and dehydration. Close monitoring of fluid intake/output and initiation of corrective measures minimizes this risk of dehydration.

  — Blood urea nitrogen (BUN) is a laboratory test of serum urea levels. Normal parameters are: 5-20 mg/dl (although findings may vary according to the laboratory equipment used).

  — Elevated BUN suggests excess protein breakdown which may occur with tissue trauma or poor excretion of urea. BUN is not specific for renal dysfunction. Other laboratory tests reflecting inadequate excretion confirm renal dysfunction. A relative elevation in BUN can occur in the presence of dehydration.

- Creatinine is another end or waste product of cellular metabolism and muscle breakdown. Creatinine production usually is fixed yielding a uniform rate throughout the day. As dietary intake does not influence creatinine production, serum levels are a good indicator of the kidney's filtration ability.

— Elevated serum creatinine levels and an abnormal BUN/creatinine ratio warrant further evaluation for possible renal dysfunction. Although findings may vary according to the laboratory equipment used, normal parameters are:

— Serum creatinine   0.5-1.5 mg/dl

— BUN/creatinine ratio   10:1-15:1

• The glomerular membrane is relatively impervious to large cells and substances. Blood cells and plasma proteins normally do not pass into the renal filtrate and tubular network. Thus, blood cells and proteins are not normally present in the urine.

— The presence of electrolytes, glucose, RBC, WBC, protein, or bacteria in the urine typically increases the urinary specific gravity. Urine osmolarity is a better indicator of renal ability to concentrate urine.

• The kidneys directly excrete some medications and illicit drugs. Other medications and drugs are metabolized by the liver and converted into inactive forms. These metabolic end products are then excreted by the kidneys. Some medications and drugs cause damage to renal tissue (nephrotoxic). Astute observation for the onset of side or toxic effects is necessary so that the health care provider can make dosage adjustments to minimize renal damage.

5. Erythropoiesis:

• Erythropoiesis refers to the production of red blood cells. The kidneys release erythropoietin in response to decreased serum oxygen levels (hypoxemia) in the blood delivered to the kidneys. In turn, erythropoietin stimulates the bone marrow to produce more red blood cells and prolongs the life of existing RBC's.

Age Variations:

1. Considerations related to the elderly:

- As an individual ages, the renal blood flow and glomerular filtration rate and numbers of functioning nephrons gradually decrease. The number of functioning nephrons decreases by approximately 30-50% with advancing years. This decrease in renal function affects an elder's capacity to compensate for changes in other body system functions.

  — Decreased numbers of functioning nephrons delay the elimination of medications in the urine. An accumulation of medications in the plasma may lead to toxic effects on other body organs.

- Glucose and bicarbonate molecules are not efficiently reabsorbed with advancing years. Sudden changes in the serum pH and circulating fluid volume may lead to serious physiological imbalances. For example, fluid loss due to diarrhea or vomiting may precipitate renal insufficiency or acute renal failure.

  — Altered glucose filtration and reabsorption often occur. Acceptable parameters for an elder are: 52-135 mm/dl.

- The renin-angiotensin-aldosterone cycle becomes less responsive to systemic changes. Diminished ability to reabsorb sodium and excrete potassium excesses results in serum electrolyte imbalances. The ability to reabsorb water and concentrate urine also decreases. Thus, the ability to adjust to intravascular changes is significantly impaired.

2. Considerations related to children:

- Critically ill children tend to retain fluid due to increased antidiuretic hormone and aldosterone secretion. Tailoring postoperative fluid administration to meet individual needs minimizes the risk for fluid overload.

- Gastroenteritis is a common cause of dehydration in infants and young children and may develop insidiously. The extracellular space in a young child contains a greater proportion of fluid than an adult. Extracellular fluid in this compartment exchanges daily and fluctuates with physiological and metabolic needs. A risk of fluid overload and/or water intoxication may occur with the rapid replacement of fluid losses.

- Non-oliguric acute renal failure (ARF) is more common in children than adults; therefore, early signs of renal impairment may go undetected.

- Children tolerate peritoneal dialysis better than hemodialysis because of the amount of blood required for the extracorporeal circuit used in hemodialysis. As children rarely experience other body system dysfunctions along with chronic renal failure (CRF), they generally are good candidates for transplantation.

Section 2: PATHOPHYSIOLOGY

1. When perfusion or blood flow to the kidneys decreases, renal ischemia occurs. The cells of the kidneys become damaged. If the ischemic state is prolonged or profound, the resulting cellular metabolic state becomes hypoxic and then anoxic. These severely damaged tissues may become necrotic and die with resulting scar formation. These areas never regain normal physiological function.

   - Tissues surrounding the site of direct damage become edematous, interfering with capillary circulation. The area of impaired renal function widens. These areas of injured and edematous tissue may recover and restore to normal physiological function.

2. **Types of renal tissue injury (pathophysiology):**

   - Acute renal failure (ARF) refers to the acute onset of renal damage and abrupt deterioration in physiological function. Acute tubular necrosis (ATN) refers to a state of acute renal failure in which death of renal tissue occurs. With prompt correction of the causative factor, ARF is reversible with restoration of normal renal function.

— Three phases of ARF occur. The characteristic of the first phase is oliguria which lasts approximately 7-21 days. The diuretic phase involves the doubling of urinary output often disproportionate to fluid intake. Renal function continues to improve. Return to a functional state may take 6-12 months (recovery phase).

• Chronic renal failure (CRF) refers to the gradual, irreversible, and progressive decline in renal function. Generally, long standing systemic pathophysiology contributes to the onset and progression of renal failure. When CRF declines to a symptomatic state, renal damage is irreversible.

— End-stage renal failure (ESRF) refers to the terminal stage of chronic renal failure which requires continuous and rigorous treatment to control the symptoms of renal dysfunction.

— Uremia and uremic syndrome are older terms associated with CRF and ESRD. These terms sometimes are used interchangeably.

3. When the function of one kidney is severely impaired, the other kidney will compensate and overall filtration is adequate. The presence of clinical manifestations and altered laboratory values associated with renal dysfunction typically do not appear until almost 75% loss of total kidney function occurs.

• Diminished renal reserve refers to marginally normal renal function which provides adequate elimination and regulatory activities under stable physiological conditions. However, a change in systemic physiological status (i.e., common cold, infection, stress) produces increased metabolic and elimination needs greater than the capability of marginally functioning kidneys. Many elderly persons have diminished renal reserve and are asymptomatic until an illness occurs.

- Renal insufficiency refers to the decline in combined renal function with only 10-25% normal activity remaining. With adherence to conservative interventions, these kidneys are able to perform sufficient physiological activity to reflect laboratory values WNL.

- Renal failure refers to the decline in combined renal function with less than 10% remaining normal activity. In this clinical situation, achieving physiological renal function requires dialysis as well as conservative interventions.

4. Several nonrenal pathophysiological conditions impair renal function. These conditions result in perfusion to the kidneys or cause direct damage to renal tissue. Tissue damage results from toxic or ischemic factors.

- Toxins to renal tissue include some medications; endotoxins from systemic infection (beta-hemolytic streptococcus); allergic reactions; some insecticides; some cleaning agents.

  — The administration of some antibiotics may precipitate loss of renal function especially in postoperative and critically ill persons. Nephrotoxicity is the consequence of accumulated high concentrations of medication in the nephrons. Examples of nephrotoxic antibiotics include aminoglycosides, gentamicin, tobramycin, kanamycin, streptomycin, penicillin, cephalosporin, cephalothin.

  — Some ACE inhibitors (captopril, enalapril) and some nonsteroidal anti-inflammatory agents may also precipitate loss of renal function.

- Factors that impair renal perfusion include: systemic shock; long-term or poorly controlled diabetes mellitus; chronic hypertension; systemic lupus; glomerulonephritis.

5. Altered electrolyte regulation:

- Potassium is an electrolyte present in most oral foods. As the body has virtually no storage capability for potassium, daily intake and regulated excretion are necessary to maintain normal serum levels.

Potassium is essential for normal electrical impulse transmission which is crucial for optimal myocardial function. Excess potassium in circulation alters impulse transmission and lethal ventricular dysrhythmias may develop.

- Normally, a proportionate balance between serum potassium and sodium ions exists. Elevated serum potassium levels generally result in decreased serum sodium levels. An abnormal serum potassium/sodium ratio alters the intracellular balance of these electrolytes. Impaired cellular function throughout the body occurs.

- With the loss of renal function, decreased vitamin D utilization occurs which decreases intestinal absorption of calcium. Normally, a proportionate balance between serum calcium and phosphate ions exists. A decrease in serum calcium levels usually triggers the release of parathyroid hormone which increases the reabsorption of calcium, excretion of phosphate and the release of calcium from the bones. This sequence of events to maintain the calcium-phosphate balance is dysfunctional when CRF exits.

  — The body attempts to hide the excess phosphate by forming crystals which are deposited in soft tissue. These deposits may occur in joints, myocardium, lungs, brain, blood vessels, and/or conjunctiva. Eventually, phosphate deposits interfere with physiological function of the affected anatomical structures.

Function   Dysfunction

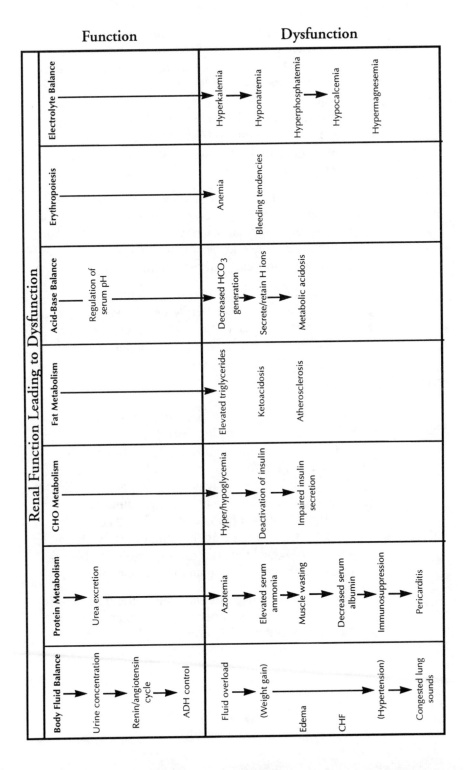

— A secondary hyperparathyroidism develops as increasing quantities of parathyroid hormone attempt to maintain normal serum calcium levels. In response to an inadequate supply of absorbed calcium from oral intake, bones provide an internal source of calcium. Eventually, bones become porous and prone to fractures. Renal osteodystrophy refers to the development of this orthopedic complication of CRF.

• Enzyme reaction, cell wall integrity and neuromuscular impulse transmission require adequate levels of magnesium. Optimal magnesium levels closely relate to other electrolyte levels. Intracellular fluid primarily contains magnesium and potassium.

— Serum imbalances of magnesium and calcium produce similar clinical manifestations. Hypermagnesemia has a depressant effect while hypomagnesemia typically produces hyperactive neuromuscular activity.

6. Altered fluid balance:

• Achieving fluid balance by regulating intake and urinary output to meet cellular need is a major function of the kidneys. When intake exceeds elimination capability, fluid retention occurs. Hypertension develops when the intravascular compartment contains excess fluid. Some intravascular fluid escapes into the interstitial compartment forming edema in the soft tissue, lung tissue, intestinal tract, nephrons, and brain. A cycle of fluid excess, leading to hypertension and increasing renal dysfunction, evolves.

• The presence of hypertension within the renal arterioles damages the semi-permeable membrane of the glomerulus. Altered filtration occurs, and renal tissue damage widens.

7. Altered metabolism of nutrients:

- Protein metabolism produces urea and creatinine as waste products which the kidneys normally remove. As excess urea and creatinine are very toxic to many body tissues, these substances must be excreted daily. When the kidneys are unable to remove sufficient quantities, the blood urea nitrogen (BUN), serum creatinine and BUN: creatinine ratio reflect the degree of accumulation in the blood. The toxic effects of the accumulation cause further renal tissue damage.

  — Urea decomposes in the gastrointestinal tract releasing ammonia (NH_3). This substance is irritating to the GI mucosa causing ulcerations and bleeding. Ammonia is also toxic to neural tissue, especially to brain cells, and can produce irreversible brain damage.

- Elevated triglyceride levels are due to increased synthesis and impaired elimination. An increased risk for atherosclerotic sequelae exists.

- Decreased serum albumin levels with normal BUN and creatinine levels suggest inadequate protein intake, malnutritional state, or protein loss in the urine. If carbohydrate or caloric intake is inadequate, natural protein stores (muscle and plasma protein) are used for energy sources and metabolic activity. Impaired healing also results.

- With the loss of renal function, uric acid excretion declines. Accumulated serum uric acid leads to the onset of gouty arthritis.

8. Altered acid-base balance (buffering capability):

- When kidneys are no longer able to appropriately respond to internal acid-base homeostasis, a state of metabolic acidosis develops. The serum pH falls and altered cellular metabolism occurs.

- Hyperkalemia often accompanies metabolic acidosis. Cells attempt to temporarily adjust to an acidotic state by accepting hydrogen in exchange for potassium within the intracellular compartment. This hydrogen-potassium exchange contributes to an elevating serum potassium level. Damaged kidneys are unable to excrete the excesses.

9. **Decreased red blood cell activity:**

- The life span of RBC's shortens and cell production decreases. A below normal RBC level results in altered oxygen carrying capacity. While oxygen supply to the circulatory system is adequate, the delivery of oxygen to the tissue level is inadequate. Tissue hypoxia results. If this situation becomes severe, altered cellular metabolism aggravates the state of metabolic acidosis.

- Chronic anemia develops from altered RBC activity and from accumulation of minute blood loss which occurs with each hemodialysis treatment. Another source of minute chronic blood loss occurs in the gastrointestinal tract due to capillary fragility and mucosal irritation.

- Bleeding tendencies accompany platelet dysfunction caused by the presence of uremic toxins (excess urea and ammonia in circulation). Skin bruising also occurs.

- Bone marrow suppression results. Iron and vitamin deficiencies develop. These situations contribute to altered hematological status.

Indications of renal dysfunction

1. Decrease in urinary output to less than 500 ml/day or less than 30 ml/hour. This decrease occurs although sufficient fluid intake to produce normal volumes of urine is present.

> If urinary output is not restored CONTACT PHYSICIAN document findings and actions.

Decision Tree for Acute Episode of Decreased Urinary Output

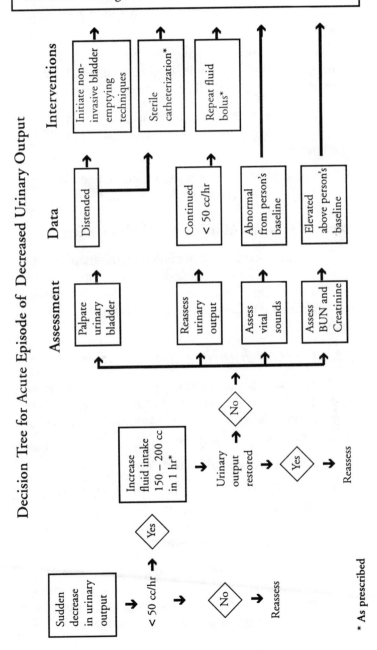

* As prescribed

- Urine analysis reveals: fixed specific gravity, presence of protein, blood cells, and possibly bacteria.

2. Evidence of body fluid excess. Clinical manifestations include: hypertension, weight gain, pitting edema, congested lung sounds.

3. Abnormal serum values include: potassium > 5.5 mEq/L; calcium < 4.5 mEq/L; phosphate > 4.5 mEq/L; magnesium > 2.5 mEq/L; sodium < 135 mEq/L.

   - Evidence of metabolic acidosis: pH; HCO_3 < 22 mEq/L. Respiratory compensation: $paCO_2$ < 35 mmHg.

4. Hematological analysis reveals chronic anemia. Hct < 35%; Hgb < 10G/dl and RBC < 4million/cm.

Section 3: MANAGEMENT AND CARE

The focus of management of clinical manifestations and facilitating renal function includes three groups of activities: (1) measures to improve renal function, (2) conservative regime of interventions, and (3) continuous and/or rigorous interventions.

Measures to Improve Renal Function

The recognition of the warning signs of impending renal dysfunction ensures the prompt initiation of measures to improve renal function, thus the likelihood of irreversible renal tissue damage diminishes.

1. Establish a baseline of fluid status:

- Since intake and output normally are balanced, an imbalance warrants further investigation. When fluid intake exceeds urine production or urinary output, renal dysfunction may exist.

- Accurate calculation of fluid intake and urinary output is required when renal dysfunction is suspected. Day-to-day calculations ("running I&O") detect continual excesses or deficits. Daily body weight is a good indicator of fluid gains or losses. A change of 2.2 pounds or 1 Kg in body weight equals a change of 1000 ml of fluid.

- Urinary specific gravity is a noninvasive test of the kidneys' ability to concentrate urine and the permeability of the glomerulus. When large cells are present in the urine, the specific gravity increases. This finding typically accompanies increased glomerular filtration rather than the ability to concentrate urine.

  — Low urine specific gravity (< 1.010) suggests dilute urine. A high urine specific gravity (> 1.030) suggests concentrated urine or the presence of large cells in the urine.

  — A fixed or unchanging specific gravity despite varying fluid intake suggests renal damage.

2. Provide adequate fluid intake to ensure adequate urine production and urinary output but not to exceed requirements for cellular activity.

   - When the urinary output is disproportionately less than the fluid intake, the bedside nurse is alert for possible renal dysfunction. When the urinary output decreases to less than 50 ml/hour, identification of the cause is essential. An hourly output below 30 ml/hour warrants prompt corrective intervention.

   - Increased fluid intake is one corrective intervention if the underlying physiological condition permits. Following the administration of a bolus of 300 cc of IV fluid in one hour, a prompt increase in urine output occurs when renal function is adequate.

     — If a fluid bolus does not result in an increase in urine output, then a diuretic may be prescribed. This group of medications selectively blocks the reabsorption of sodium and water from the renal tubules producing an increase in urinary output. With a sudden elimination of urine, there is a comparable decrease in intravascular volume. Orthostatic hypotension with an increased risk for falling may occur, especially in an elderly person.

— Electrolytes, especially sodium and potassium, are typically excreted along with the excess fluid or urine. Assessment of clinical manifestations and laboratory values for lowered values prevent secondary (iatrogenic) complications.

3. Restore serum potassium values to normal parameters Electrolyte values are usually abnormal when renal dysfunction occurs. Elevated serum potassium levels result in the most serious consequences and require prompt correction. Potassium is required for effective electrical impulse transmission in muscles, including the myocardium. When serum levels rise, QRS complexes widen, P waves flatten and disappear. Ventricular tachycardia, ventricular fibrillation, or asystole may occur.

- Serum potassium levels 6.0 mEq/L require prompt removal of excess serum potassium to minimize the risk of a lethal dysrhythmia.

  — IV administration of hypertonic glucose with insulin temporarily moves the excess potassium from the serum into the cells.

  — IV administration of calcium temporarily counteracts the adverse effects that excess potassium has on the myocardium. The risk for ventricular dysrhythmias diminishes.

  — Oral or rectal administration of sodium polystyrene sulfonate (Kayexalate) binds with potassium in the large intestine for excretion. Depending upon the dosage and extent of use, diarrhea often occurs.

  — Dialysis is the most effective treatment for achieving electrolyte and fluid balance when renal dysfunction is present.

Arterial Blood Gas (ABG) Analysis

Data provided by one or a series of ABG values increase the understanding of appropriate nursing interventions and medical management of individuals with acute metabolic conditions. This unit addresses the changes in the acid-base balance related to metabolic/renal dysfunction and respiratory compensation. Refer to Unit 2 for additional discussion of underlying respiratory causes for acid-base imbalances.

The following three steps provide pertinent data from a given ABG:

Step 1: Look at the pH to determine the general acid-base state.

- Normal parameters (WNL) for pH: 7.35-7.45

- If the pH is below 7.35, the acid-base imbalance is acidosis.

- If the pH is above 7.45, the acid-base imbalance is alkalosis.

Step 2: Look at the $paCO_2$ and HCO_3 values to determine the type of acid-base imbalance due to metabolic/renal pathophysiology.

- Normal parameters (WNL) for HCO_3 are: 22-26 mEq/L (although findings may vary according to the laboratory equipment used).

- If the HCO_3 value is below 22 mEq/L and the pH is below 7.35, then the primary acid-base imbalance is metabolic acidosis.

- If the HCO_3 value is above 26 mEq/L and the pH is above 7.46, then the primary acid-base imbalance is metabolic alkalosis.

- With abnormal HCO_3 values and $paCO_2$ values WNL, the acid-base imbalance is UNCOMPENSAT-ED metabolic acidosis or alkalosis.

Step 3: Look at the $paCO_2$ to determine the degree of compensation provided by the respiratory system.

- The respiratory system responds quickly, often within minutes, to a metabolic acid-base imbalance. Carbon dioxide is either retained with shallower and slower respirations to lower the pH toward 7.45 or exhaled with rapid, deep respirations to increase the pH toward 7.35.

- Normal parameters for $paCO_2$ are: 35-45 mmHg (although findings may vary according to the laboratory equipment used).

- When metabolic acidosis is present (HCO_3 mEq/L and pH is below 7.35), a gradual fall in the $paCO_2$ below the normal parameter (35 mmHg) reflects respiratory compensation. Rapid, deep respirations "blow off" carbon dioxide which act as an acid reducing respiratory compensatory state. The pH will rise toward normal (7.35). This acid-base imbalance is called COMPENSATING metabolic acidosis.

  — A similar but reverse pattern of compensation occurs with a primary metabolic alkalotic state.

- When the respiratory compensation balances the metabolic imbalance, the pH is WNL. A balance between a primary metabolic imbalance and respiratory compensation is called COMPENSATED metabolic acidosis or alkalosis.

- When metabolic acidosis and respiratory acidosis are present at the same time, a combined acidotic state is present. This serious imbalance is associated with a rapidly falling pH. If uncorrected, respiratory and cardiac arrest are imminent and the mortality rate is high.

Focused Bedside Assessment

The following is a guideline of expected data from a head-to-toe assessment of an adult experiencing poorly controlled, chronic renal failure and the associated body system involvement. Pathophysiological problems not related to chronic renal failure and the systemic effects are not included.

- **General Appearance:** malaise; sallow, yellowish skin color; weak and fatigued; subnormal body temperature; dry, brittle hair; periorbital edema.

- **Neurological Status:** lethargy; confusion; irritability; headache; possible seizure activity; blurred vision.

- **Cardiac/Circulatory Status:** fluid overload with elevated CVP and PCWP; hypertension; pericardial effusion; palpitations; at risk for ventricular dysrhythmias; interstitial edema; bounding peripheral pulses; anemia.

- **Respiratory Status:** dyspnea; labored breathing; orthopnea; congested lung sounds; pleural effusion; Kussmaul respirations if severely acidotic.

- **Abdominal (GI) Status:** nausea with vomiting; anorexia; gastritis; stomatitis; epigastric pain; belching with reflux; metallic taste; halitosis; thirst; flank or groin pain.

- **Urinary Elimination Status:** progressive decrease in urinary output in spite of fluid intake; unchanging (fixed) urinary specific gravity despite fluid intake; foul smelling urine; oliguria to anuria; dysuria, nocturia, hematuria, proteinuria, or pyuria.

- **Extremities:** dependent, pitting edema; paresthesia in the feet; motor weakness; pallor; dry, itchy skin; muscle twitching (restless leg syndrome); nocturnal leg cramps; petechiae and/or ecchymoses; brittle often discolored nails.

- When the individual is turned to his/her side, the nurse would expect to find: sacral edema if on bedrest; petechiae and/or ecchymoses.

If additional data are observed, a more detailed assessment of the involved body system is required. Additional areas of physiological dysfunction may be present and confound the present renal problem.

Conservative Regime of Interventions:

1. Control of underlying pathophysiological conditions is essential in slowing the progression of renal tissue damage. Collaboration between health care providers and the individual to control the underlying condition increases the success of the management plan. Without commitment of the individual to the plan of care, conservative management has limited success.

   - Diabetes mellitus and essential hypertension are the two most common underlying conditions associated with the development of chronic renal failure. Control of these conditions delays the onset of renal complications. However, many persons do not accept the responsibility for adhering to their medical plan of care, and the insidious development of renal failure occurs.

2. **Psychosocial support:**

   - Conservative measures involve major changes in lifestyle including marked fluid and dietary restriction and numerous daily medications. Most persons benefit from counseling to aid in their adjustment to this chronic condition. The stages of adjustment include: "honeymoon" stage, disenchantment/discouragement, and the stage of adaptation.

     — The honeymoon stage begins when the person begins conservative management or dialysis treatments. The person begins to physically feel better. His or her outlook improves and the person no longer experiences the feeling of imminent death. This stage typically lasts 6 weeks to 6 months.

     — The period of disenchantment and discouragement begins when the person realizes that he/she will depend upon this involved medical regime for the rest of his/her life. Expressions of anger, depression, helplessness, or hopelessness are common. Financial strains and changes in family dynamics add to the psychosocial aspects on long-term treatment. Most persons experience this period for 3-12 months; however, some persons may remain at varying degrees of denial or helplessness for longer periods of time.

— During the stage of adaptation, the person begins to accept the illness as an extension of life. With the advances in techniques and medications, the occurrence of complications continues to decrease. Depending upon the age of onset, life expectancy, with responsible management, is 20 years or longer.

3. **Nutritional therapy** focuses on achieving optimal nutritional status, minimizing uremic toxicity and preventing protein catabolism.

   • A renal diet includes restriction of protein, fluid, sodium, potassium and phosphate while maintaining adequate caloric intake. This dietary plan may also include diabetic requirements.

   — Protein intake equals cellular need. Excess protein results in increased quantities of urea and creatinine in circulation which cannot be sufficiently excreted by the damaged kidneys. Periodic creatinine clearance testing determines adjustments in the daily protein intake appropriate for the current renal status.

   — The administration of amino acids or TPN during dialysis treatments supplements nutritional needs when oral intake is inadequate. By providing these nutrients during dialysis, the excess fluid associated with TPN can be removed and only the nutrients remain in circulation.

   — The amount of fluid permitted each day equals urinary output plus 500 ml for insensible loss. Body weight and blood pressure are valuable guides in determining fluid status. Fluid intake includes liquids and food sources with high liquid content. The person fills a container each morning with the required daily fluid volume. This volume of fluid includes all beverages and fluid for taking medications.

— Sodium restriction minimizes water retention, weight gain, and hypertension. Most commercially prepared foods contain sodium seasoning.

— Potassium restriction minimizes excesses that trigger cardiac dysrhythmias. Most foods contain potassium, especially many fresh fruits and organ meats.

— Phosphate restriction minimizes phosphate accumulations which accompany hypocalcemia and bone changes. Foods high in phosphate also tend to be good protein sources.

• Adequate caloric intake minimizes the use of protein stores as a source of energy and cellular metabolism. When the body uses its natural protein stores, a state of negative nitrogen balance occurs and muscle wasting develops.

— The liberal use of tart-flavored hard candy provides a source of calories and also appeases the constant feeling of a dry mouth. Meticulous mouth care minimizes the onset of dental caries and gingival irritation from the presence of sugars on the teeth.

• Vitamin supplements provide an added source when dietary restrictions may not provide sufficient quantities. Sufficient quantities of vitamin D, iron and folic acid are often difficult to acquire by diet alone.

4. Medication regime:

• Stool softeners or laxatives counteract the occurrence of constipation which develops secondarily to limited fluid intake and antacid administration.

- Diuretics promote fluid excretion and reduce hypertension. Potassium excreting agents are acceptable since elevated potassium levels may also occur.

- Hematological agents increase RBC production. Examples include folic acid, ferrous sulfate, ferrous gluconate, Imferon.

  — Synthetic erythropoietin (Epogen) is now available for intramuscular administration to correct severe and prolonged anemia which often accompanies CRF.

- Vitamin D enhances calcium absorption from the GI tract. Examples include Rocaltrol.

- Calcium supplements minimize calcium loss from bones and maintain optimal serum levels. Examples include titralac, calcium carbonate, or calcium gluconate.

- Phosphate binding antacids bind with dietary phosphorus in the GI tract to minimize absorption into the blood. When taken with meals, these antacids have optimal binding effects with dietary phosphate. Desirable antacids do not contain aluminum, magnesium or sodium which could lead to serum excesses. Examples of desirable phosphate binding antacids are Amphojel, Basaljel, AlternaGel.

- Allopurinol facilitates the excretion of uric acid molecules and minimizes the formation of uric acid crystals.

- Supplemental insulin ("sliding scale") is often required for most critically ill persons with renal failure because hyperglycemia is common even in non-diabetic persons.

- A variety of anti-hypertensive agents are prescribed to control a pre-existing hypertensive state. As dialysis treatment removes some of these medications, scheduling the times of administration in coordination with the dialysis treatment results in effective blood pressure management. Doses of these medications on days between dialysis treatments may require adjustment because of accumulated effects resulting from minimal excretion.

Continuous and/or rigorous interventions:

One specific treatment modality for renal failure is dialysis — a mechanical means for maintaining fluid and electrolytes within acceptable parameters. Dialysis is the treatment of choice when the kidneys fail to respond to fluid challenges, diuretic administration, and electrolyte regulation. Typically, an individual experiencing the oliguric/anuric stage of ARF for more than 4-5 days requires temporary dialysis. Individuals experiencing chronic renal failure with less than 25% remaining renal function require long-term dialysis.

Dialysis is a process that permits the diffusion or movement of fluids and particles across a semi-permeable membrane. The particles manipulated include potassium, sodium, calcium, phosphate, and bicarbonate. This artificial process resembles the functioning of a normal nephron. Dialysis does not correct the renal dysfunction or the pathology caused by renal tissue damage; it only corrects fluid, electrolyte, and acid-base imbalances. Discussion of three types of dialysis modalities includes hemodialysis, continuous arteriovenous hemofiltration, and peritoneal dialysis. In addition, renal transplantation is the desired treatment modality for persons who meet selected criteria. These modalities have decreased the mortality associated with ARF and increased the quality of life and longevity of life for persons with ESRD.

There are some unique considerations regarding medication therapy and dialysis. First, delayed metabolism and excretion of some medications between dialysis treatments may lead to accumulated quantities circulating in the blood. Occurrence of side or toxic effects increases with usual, normal doses. Second, many drugs cross the semi-permeable membrane of the dialyzer leading to less than therapeutic levels following a dialysis treatment.

1. Hemodialysis:

- Hemodialysis requires direct vascular access. The subclavian and femoral vessels are the common access sites for short-term treatments via the insertion of a central catheter. The surgical creation of internal arteriovenous fistula, shunt, or graft provides permanent access for long-term treatment.

- The process of hemodialysis involves pumping venous blood from the person via his or her venous access through tubing and dialyzer. Blood returns to the person's circulatory system via the arterial access. Blood circulates through this closed system which regulates the rate of fluid and electrolyte exchange by varying the flow rates and pressures.

- Diffusion or movement of fluid and particles occurs in the dialyzer which contains thousands of tubes which are only one-cell in diameter. The person's blood passes through these tiny tubes which are surrounded by a solution (dialysate). The walls of the tubes act as semi-permeable membrane allowing only small particles to move from the blood into the dialysate. Due to a constant flow of dialysate, diffused particles are carried away in other tubing which empties in a fluid waste system.

  — A dialyzer is sometimes called an artificial kidney.

- Small particles that move into the dialysate include potassium, creatinine, urea, uric acid, and water molecules. Larger particles such as proteins, blood cells, and bacteria do not cross the dialyzer membrane and remain in the person's blood. The concentration of particles in the person's blood and the composition of the dialysate controls the degree of fluid and particle exchange.

  — When only excess potassium is removed from a person's blood, the dialysate contains a minimal concentration of potassium.

— For persons with a seriously low pH due to low serum bicarbonate levels, the use of a dialysate with bicarbonate molecules is appropriate.

— The dialysate typically includes 133-145 mEq/L of sodium which is the normal serum level. Only excess sodium in a person's blood moves into the dialysate.

• Hemodialysis provides rapid and efficient removal of excess water and particles from acute poisoning and acute renal failure. This modality requires vascular access and heparin to maintain the patency of lines. Very young and elderly persons generally experience hemodynamic instability during treatment.

• Specific care measures associated with hemodialysis include:

— Hemodialysis treatments 2-3 times per week maintain optimal fluid and electrolyte balance for persons with ESRD. Accurate measurements of body weight prior to dialysis and comparison to an individual's "dry weight" determines the amount of fluid removed during a treatment. Frequent assessment of blood pressure, coagulation and cardiac rhythm during treatment provides data on possible hemodynamic and cardiac side effects.

— If the person has a central line for hemodialysis access, the ports generally are not used for any other purpose. The rationale is to ensure a patent access for treatment. Between treatments, the ports are capped and the lines contain a heparinized solution. The care of the insertion site is similar to other central line care measures.

— The surgical creation of an arteriovenous fistula typically resembles a side-to-side anastomosis between an artery and vein. The fistula requires approximately 4-6 weeks to heal sufficiently to allow for insertion of the access needles. During the healing phase, the site (especially the arm) often appears edematous. Elevation of the site relieves some of the vascular congestion.

— The surgical placement of a synthetic graft between an artery and vein is a common procedure for creating permanent access. Some postoperative edema is common.

— During the healing phase, assessment of the quality of circulation and patency of the fistula or graft are essential. The palpation of a thrill or auscultation of a bruit over the fistula or graft indicates patency. The turbulence of blood flow at the site results from the mixing of arterial and venous blood.

— Assessment of peripheral circulation distal to the site is essential. Compression by edematous soft tissue or occlusion of the fistula or graft may occur. Peripheral pulses distal to the fistula or graft should be equal to the unaffected extremity. The presence of tingling or loss of sensation may indicate neurological impairment. Circulation distal to the site may become impaired ("steal syndrome").

— Avoid obtaining blood pressure assessments and blood samples from the extremity with a fistula or graft. These procedures may interfere with the patency or inadvertently damage the fistula or graft. The use of constricting clothing or jewelry is avoided for the same reason.

2. Continuous Arteriovenous Hemofiltration (CAVH) is a relatively new dialysis modality for acute, hemodynamically unstable clinical conditions. Its use is primarily in critical care settings.

Continuous Arteriovenous Hemofiltration

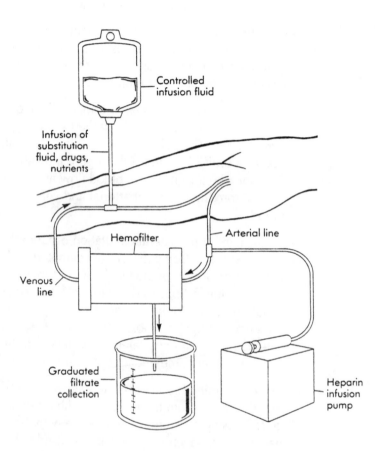

Controlled infusion fluid

Infusion of substitution fluid, drugs, nutrients

Hemofilter

Arterial line

Venous line

Graduated filtrate collection

Heparin infusion pump

Janet-Beth McCann Flynn and Nancy Purdue Bruce.
Introduction to Critical Care Skills, Mosby-Year Book, 1993.
Reprinted by permission.

- With this modality, the person's blood enters the CAVH system via a temporary vascular access. The femoral artery and vein are the common access sites. The person's own blood pressure determines the flow rate through the system. The volume of blood in the CAVH system at any one time is much less compared to a hemodialysis system.

— Blood flows through a hemofilter which contains a semi-permeable membrane. The hemofilter resembles a dialyzer and facilitates diffusion in a similar manner. Differences in pressures and solute concentration between the person's blood and filtrate solution determines the rate of water and particle movement. The rate of diffusion is much slower and less efficient as compared to hemodialysis.

• Because CAVH is slow and less blood circulates in the system, persons who are physiologically unstable tolerate this treatment with fewer side effects than those on hemodialysis. The removal of excess fluid, electrolyte, and toxic substances is effective.

3. **Peritoneal Dialysis** (PD) uses the person's own peritoneal lining and vasculature as the semipermeable membrane. As with other forms of dialysis, this system is closed and sterile. Dialyzing solution flows by gravity into the peritoneal cavity through a surgically placed catheter. The solution remains in the peritoneal cavity for a designated period of time to allow for movement of water and particles from the blood into the dialyzing solution. The dialyzing solution with additional water and particles, drain from the cavity by gravity.

• Continuous ambulatory peritoneal dialysis (CAPD) is a variation of peritoneal dialysis used in the management of CRF. This modality is an in-home, self-care technique which persons learn in a 2-3 week training period.

— CAPD involves the instillation of sterile solution and drainage of peritoneal fluid every four hours. After instillation, the empty solution bag and tubing remains attached to the flow catheter but is folded and secured to the abdomen. The person

resumes normal daily activities between instillation and drainage. In the evening, dialysate fluid
remains in the peritoneal cavity overnight. This
four cycle pattern maintains normal fluid and
electrolyte balance for responsible persons with
CRF.

— Infection and peritonitis are complications associated with peritoneal dialysis. Annoying problems
include abdominal distention, hernia formation,
and constipation due to pressure on the large
intestine and rectum, and poor appetite or indi-
gestion due to pressure on the stomach.

• Specific care measures associated with peritoneal
dialysis include:

— Because of the ever-present risk of acquired infection, especially peritonitis, the inside of all tubing
and connection ports must remain sterile.
Dialysate solution is also sterile. Meticulous handwashing and aseptic technique are the best preventive measures.

— Dialysate return normally appears clear and pale
— straw colored. Cloudy appearance is an early
indicator of possible infection. This change in the
appearance of the dialysate return flow typically
precedes other clinical manifestations of infection,
such as abdominal pain or fever.

4. Transplantation:

• Renal transplantation is the treatment of choice for
children and adults with no other pathophysiological
problems. Recent development of immunosuppressive medications decreased the risk of complications
and increased life expectancy of persons with CRF.
Post-transplant lifestyle includes continual medication and modified dietary regime without dialysis.

— Transplantation is not a cure for renal failure but another treatment modality for selected persons.

- Presurgical preparation includes extensive physical and psychosocial evaluation. A series of tissue-matching tests determine optimal compatibility with minimal risk of rejection. Transplanted kidneys come from either living, related donor or heartbeating cadaver donor. (Refer to Unit 1 for additional information on outcomes of brain death and criteria for organ/tissue donation.)

  — Actual implantation involves surgical placement of the donor kidney into a recipient within 72 hours of removal from the donor. Renal artery, vein, and ureter are surgically attached adjacent to existing structures.

  — Urine production from the donor kidney generally occurs within 2-3 days of implantation. Temporary dialysis may be required until adequate renal function resumes in the transplanted kidney.

- Immunosuppressive therapy after surgery delays the onset of rejection. Medications include corticosteroids (Prednisone), purine analogues (azathioprine/Imuran), antilymphocyte globulin, and cyclosporine (Sandimmune).

- Signs of rejection include: fluid retention, hypertension, oliguria, temperature elevation, weight gain, malaise, and elevated lab values (BUN, potassium, and creatinine). These clinical signs resemble the onset of renal failure. Prompt and aggressive treatment can reverse this response and restore renal function.

Unit 7

Care of Individuals with High Acuity Digestive and/or Metabolic Conditions

T his unit addresses a variety of high acuity digestive and/or metabolic conditions associated with dysfunction of the gastrointestinal tract, liver, and pancreas. Information presented here includes the effects of disrupted physiological function on other body systems. Persons with high acuity digestive and/or metabolic conditions traditionally were cared for on critical care units. As the trends in health care shift to ambulatory, extended, and home health settings, the principles of high acuity nursing care and related nursing interventions will extend beyond the walls of the traditional acute care hospital.

An understanding of general medical-surgical nursing care of digestive and metabolic conditions provides the basis for the information presented in this unit. Prerequisite understanding includes basic normal anatomical and physiological considerations of the digestive and metabolic systems, physiological response to hormones and enzymes, normal gastrointestinal activity and elimination, as well as interventions which will improve physiological function. The extension, elaboration, and refinement of these concepts provide the foundation for the nursing care of high acuity digestive and metabolic conditions.

Section 1: REVIEW AND OVERVIEW

The structures of the digestive and metabolic systems provide an effective and efficient process for nutrient and fluid intake which are metabolized for energy and tissue building. The digestive and renal systems dispose of or eliminate unused substances and the end products of metabolism.

Anatomical Considerations

1. Gastrointestinal (GI) tract:

- The GI tract is a hollow tube that connects the oral cavity, esophagus, stomach, small intestine, and large intestine (colon) with the rectum. Ingested food and liquids pass through this tube system and undergo varying digestive changes. The small intestine and colon absorb nutritive substances and liquids. The elimination of undigested and unabsorbed substances typically occurs daily as feces.

- Large quantities of digestive secretions facilitate the digestive process.

  — The cells in the stomach wall produce about 1500-3000 ml of gastric secretions daily in response to ingested food. These secretions include hydrochloric acid, pepsin, intrinsic factor, and histamine. Gastric secretions are very acidic.

  — The cells in the small intestinal wall produce about 3000 ml of intestinal secretions daily. These secretions include digestive enzymes from the pancreas (amylase, lipase, trypsin), and bile from the liver and gall bladder. Intestinal secretions are very alkaline.

2. Liver and gall bladder:

- The liver is the largest internal organ in the body and is located under the right side of the diaphragm. Its metabolic functions require large quantities of blood.

The heart delivers approximately 800-1500 ml or 13-25% of the cardiac output to the liver per minute via the hepatic artery. The portal vein receives approximately 1000-1200 ml of deoxygenated blood per minute from the vasculature of the abdominal cavity.

— Arterial blood, filtered through the liver, and venous blood flow from the gastrointestinal tract form the hepatic venous blood supply. Portal system also refers to the venous blood flow through the liver.

• The gall bladder is a small storage sac located between the liver and the small intestine. The liver produces bile to aid in the digestion of fat. The hepatic duct carries the bile from the liver for storage in the gall bladder. In response to the presence of fat in the stomach and duodenum, the gall bladder releases bile into the duodenum via the common bile duct. The sphincter of Oddi controls the flow of bile into the duodenum.

3. Pancreas:

• The pancreas lies deep in the abdomen. Its head lies within the curve of the duodenum, and its tail lies behind the stomach and extends to the spleen in the upper left quadrant of the abdomen.

— Exocrine cells refers to cells which excrete digestive enzymes that flow into the duodenum. These enzymes and the bile flow into the duodenum through the ampulla of Vater.

— Endocrine cells refers to the Islet of Langerhans cells which secrete insulin and glucagon into the blood stream.

Normal Physiological Considerations

1. Gastrointestinal (GI) tract:

• The rate of peristalsis is approximately three waves per minute. The volume, osmotic pressure, and chemical composition of stomach contents affect the motility rate. For example, the high caloric content of the ingested food slows gastric peristalsis and delays the emptying time.

— The acidity of gastric secretions enhances pepsin activity and protein digestion. This acidic environment also inhibits bacterial growth.

• The majority of digestion and absorption of nutrients occurs in the duodenum. Bile, pancreatic enzymes, and intestinal enzymes enhance this process. Absorption of vitamins and minerals also occurs in the small intestine. Fat-soluble vitamins (A, D, E, and K) require bile for adequate absorption. Because some vitamins (B complex, C, and folic acid) are water-soluble, they are readily absorbed. For adequate absorption, vitamin B_{12} (cobalamine) requires intrinsic factor, which is secreted from the wall of the stomach.

— Chyme, or intestinal contents, usually moves through the small intestine in 3-10 hours. A "peristaltic rush" is an episode of hyperperistalsis which may occur as an attempt to quickly move potentially harmful substances through the tract. High carbohydrate intake on an empty stomach may produce a similar response —"gastrocolic reflex."

• The rate of movement of chyme through the large intestine determines water and electrolyte absorption. Decreased peristaltic rate contributes to constipation.

• The normal bacterial flora of the large intestine includes Escherichia coli and Streptococci. These micro-organisms participate in carbohydrate and lipid metabolism. Decreased peristalsis may lead to bacterial overpopulation and malabsorption of vitamins and nutrients.

— A damaged or injured intestinal wall may lead to leakage of contents and bacteria into surrounding tissue which produces a very irritating or infectious process (peritonitis).

2. Liver:

- To perform, the liver requires large quantities of venous and arterial blood for its multiple metabolic functions. More than 400 physiological functions occur within the liver. These functions cluster into three categories: storage, protection, and metabolism.

- The liver stores many nutrients from dietary intake for release as cellular needs arise. These nutrients include minerals, vitamins, and glucagon.

  — The liver also controls hepatic vascular volumes as a response to systemic circulatory changes. Pooling or release of arterial or venous blood flow within the liver aids in maintaining circulatory homeostasis.

  — The liver synthesizes and stores clotting factors (prothrombin, fibrinogen). Vitamin K is necessary to synthesize coagulation factors in the liver which participate in the clotting process.

- The protective functions of the liver include removing bacteria and harmful substances and recycling of RBC's.

  — Kupffer cells act as master filters removing bacteria and foreign particles from the portal (venous) blood. The liver alters the toxicity of many substances thereby preventing the accumulation of substances in circulation and minimizing potentially adverse effects to other organs and tissues.

  — The liver plays an active role in the breakdown and recycling of aged red blood cells. The first step in recycling red blood cells involves the separation of hemoglobin into its components by macrophages in the spleen and liver (heme and globin).

— Iron is one substance separated from the heme component. The liver stores iron until the bone marrow uses it to produce new RBC's. Biliverdin is a second substance separated from the heme by an interaction with enzymes. Once converted, biliverdin binds with albumin in the plasma and becomes fat-soluble. Unconjugated bilirubin or free bilirubin refers to this step in the metabolic sequence.

— When unconjugated bilirubin circulates through the liver, it joins with glucuronic acid to form con-jugated (direct) bilirubin, which is water-soluble. The conversion from a fat-soluble substance into a water-soluble substance permits excretion via the bile.

— Once conjugated, (direct) bilirubin reaches the large intestine where intestinal bacteria facilitate its conversion to urobilinogen. The kidneys excrete the majority of the urobilinogen in the urine with only a small amount eliminated in feces.

• The metabolic functions of the liver include the breakdown of amino acids and fatty acids into forms utilized by cells. The liver converts ammonia, an end-product of protein metabolism, into a less harm-ful substance (urea) for elimination. The metabolism of triglycerides occurs within the liver.

— The liver synthesizes plasma proteins (albumin, globulin). Normal serum values provide a fluid holding function and maintain intravascular fluid volume and blood pressure. The oncotic pressure capability of plasma proteins also regulates the fluid volume within the interstitial space. Oncotic pressure provides a counterbalance for the hydro-static pressure exerted by arterial blood flow and arterial blood pressure.

— The conversion of glucose to glycogen for storage and the conversion from glycogen to glucose for cellular energy occurs within the liver. Gluconeogenesis, the formation of glycogen from non-carbohydrate sources such as amino or fatty acids, also occurs in the liver in the presence of low carbohydrate intake or starvation.

3. Pancreas:

- The pancreas has two major physiological functional units. The exocrine unit includes the cells and ducts to secrete and deliver enzymes and alkaline fluids to the duodenum for digestive purposes. The endocrine unit includes the Islet (beta) cells which are located throughout this gland. These cells secrete glucagon and insulin into the general blood circulation to regulate carbohydrate, protein, and fat metabolism.

- Pancreatic enzymes facilitate digestion in the duodenum. Trypsin is a protein-digesting enzyme. Amylase is a carbohydrate-digesting enzyme. Lipase is a fat-digesting enzyme. These enzymes are alkaline and create the optimal environment for digestion and absorption. The presence of ingested food and liquids in the stomach stimulates pancreatic enzyme production and flow rate. These enzymes flow through a duct system and pass into the duodenum.

  — The sphincter of Oddi at the ampulla of Vater closes during periods of nondigestion. Bile becomes concentrated and the gall bladder stores the accumulated bile for future use. In response to presence of fatty food substances in the stomach and duodenum, the sphincter relaxes permitting the flow of bile through the ampulla of Vater into the duodenum.

  — Insulin converts nutrients to their simplest chemical structure for cellular metabolism. In contrast, glucagon converts nutrients into more complex forms for storage and later use.

Age Variations

1. Considerations related to the elderly:

- Peristalsis decreases and acid-base content of secretions becomes more neutral. Digestion of ingested food and absorption of nutrients slows. Intolerance of dietary fat intake results from decreased lipase and more concentrated bile.

- Metabolism and detoxification of medications slow and result in increased serum levels. The risk of drug interaction and side effects increases.

- The Islet cells of the pancreas tend to decrease in effective insulin production. The incidence of glucose intolerance and episodic hyperglycemia increases with aging. Blood glucose levels remain elevated slightly longer compared to younger adults. Non-insulin dependent diabetes mellitus (NIDDM) is a common chronic condition among the elderly.

2. Considerations related to infants and children:

The physiology of normal anatomical structures of children is very similar to adults. Congenital anomalies contribute to altered physiology.

Section 2: PATHOPHYSIOLOGY

1. Liver:

- Hepatic dysfunction may be acute or chronic. Hepatic cells are capable of remarkable healing because of their capacity to regenerate. Healing generally occurs within 3-4 months of an acute episode. However, repeated inflammatory episodes result in fibrotic replacement of damaged hepatic tissue. This fibrotic replacement tissue resembles scar formation of other body tissue and does not function as normal, healthy hepatic tissue.

- Cirrhosis refers to an end-stage process in which irreversible cellular destruction, fibrotic tissue replacement, or ineffective liver tissue is present. This condition is a reaction to severe and often repeated hepatic inflammation and necrosis. The cause may be repeated infections (hepatitis) or ingestion of hepatotoxic substances (alcohol, illicit drugs, or other toxic substances).

- Portal hypertension refers to: (1) increased venous congestion within the liver or (2) increased vascular pressure within the portal vein which normally transports venous blood from the intestines to the liver. With the subsequent backup or congestion in the portal vein, collateral circulation develops to form a by-pass around congested hepatic tissue.

  — Collateral circulation or by-pass circulation develops in the gastric and esophageal veins. Increased venous volume distends these normally small vessels. With prolonged distention, varicose veins (varices) develop which may bleed or rupture producing varying degrees of bleeding in the stomach or esophagus.

  — Congestion within the venous system also leads to the development of enlarged vessels beneath the skin surface of the abdomen, especially surrounding the umbilicus (caput medusae). Distention of rectal veins leads to the development of hemorrhoids.

- Congestion within the gastrointestinal venous system contributes to fluid retention within the interstitial space. Eventually, accumulated fluid pressure leads to fluid movement into the peritoneal cavity (ascites). Third-spacing refers to the disproportionate accumulation of fluid in the extravascular compartment.

  — Other factors which contribute to the development of ascites include low serum plasma protein and low serum sodium levels. An enlarged liver and distended abdomen (ascites) raises the diaphragm and contributes to impaired respiratory function.

- Blockage of the flow of bile from the liver into the biliary tract often leads to jaundice. Bile and the products of RBC recycling accumulate in the liver. Due to differences in pressure gradients, some bilirubin moves into the blood producing a yellowish color in the skin and sclera of the eyes.

  — Excess amounts of conjugated (direct) bilirubin, which is fat-soluble, may accumulate in the adipose tissue or the white matter of the neurological system. Prolonged and/or severe hyperbilirubinemia may lead to neural deposits and brain damage (asterixis). Although values may vary with the laboratory equipment used, conjugated (direct) bilirubin normally does not exceed 1 mg/dl.

- Inadequate protein metabolism results in decreased production of several protein substances which affect optimal body system function. With a decrease in serum albumin, a decrease in fluid movement from the interstitial space to the vascular space occurs and contributes to interstitial edema and ascites.

  — Due to a decrease in the production of fibrinogen, prothrombin and other clotting factors, the risk of impaired blood coagulation increases.

  — A decrease in immunoglobulins (IgA) and Kupffer cell activity increases the risk for secondary and nosocomial infections and delayed healing.

- One of the end products of protein metabolism is ammonia. The liver normally converts ammonia to a less toxic substance (urea), which is normally excreted by the kidneys. With liver dysfunction, ammonia accumulates in the blood. Ammonia is very toxic to the nervous system producing irreversible brain damage (hepatic encephalopathy).

Function   Dysfunction

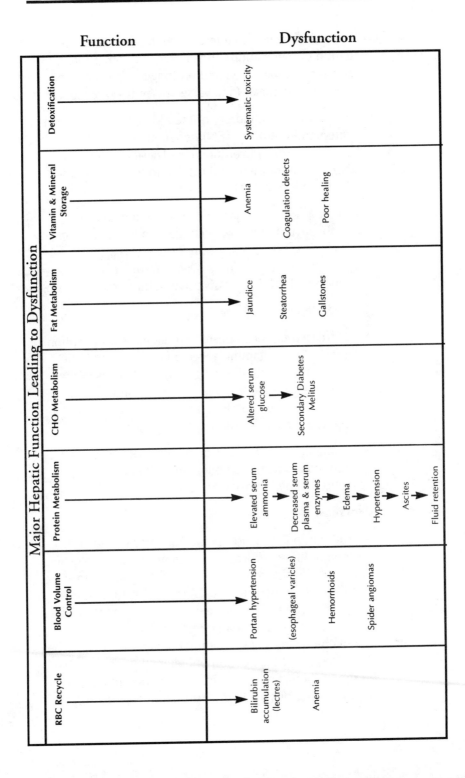

Major Hepatic Function Leading to Dysfunction

Function	Dysfunction
RBC Recycle	Bilirubin accumulation (lectres) → Anemia
Blood Volume Control	Portan hypertension (esophageal varicies) → Hemorrhoids → Spider angiomas
Protein Metabolism	Elevated serum ammonia → Decreased serum plasma & serum enzymes → Edema → Hypertension → Ascites → Fluid retention
CHO Metabolism	Altered serum glucose → Secondary Diabetes Melitus
Fat Metabolism	Jaundice → Steatorrhea → Gallstones
Vitamin & Mineral Storage	Anemia → Coagulation defects → Poor healing
Detoxification	Systematic toxicity

- Liver dysfunction interferes with the normal detoxification of medication, illicit drugs, and other foreign substances. Increased and prolonged effects of medications often lead to adverse and/or toxic reactions.

- Infants, young children, or the elderly receiving total parenteral nutrition (TPN) frequently demonstrate abnormalities in liver function. These abnormalities usually are transient and resolve following the discontinuation of TPN.

  — The presence of jaundice usually indicates obstructed bile flow secondary to hepatocellular fibrosis, bile proliferation, or bile stasis. Some degree of fibrosis may persist despite discontinuation of TPN. Progressive liver failure may develop.

2. Gallbladder:

- Decreased fat metabolism and decreased absorption of fat-soluble vitamins develop from impaired bile flow to the intestine. Undigested fat appears in the stool (steatorrhea). Decreased availability of vitamin K, a fat soluble vitamin, leads to delayed blood clotting and increased soft tissue bruising.

- An infection in the liver or systemic dehydration may produce concentrated bile. The risk of bile stone formation (cholelithiasis) increases.

3. Pancreas:

- With an inflammation of the pancreas (pancreatitis), impaired flow of digestive enzymes into the intestine occurs. Persistent stimulation of the pancreas to excrete enzymes in the presence of obstructed flow results in an enzymatic reaction with normal pancreatic tissue. A state of autodigestion develops in which enzymes act on normal pancreatic tissue. The subsequent exacerbation of inflamed pancreatic tissue furthers the mechanical obstruction of enzyme flow. A vicious cycle of obstruction, enzymatic response, autodigestion, and inflammation develops and can lead to fatty necrosis of the pancreas.

- With decreased production or noninflammatory pancreatic dysfunction, digestive enzymes do not flow into the duodenum in sufficient quantities. Impaired breakdown of dietary protein, fat, and carbohydrate occurs. Dietary fat passes through the gastrointestinal tract undigested and unabsorbed. Malabsorption of fat produces steatorrhea which is frequent, pale, bulky, frothy, foul-smelling stool. Malabsorption of protein and carbohydrate do not produce characteristic changes in elimination.

- Impaired functioning of the beta cells of the pancreatic Islets of Langerhans produces the condition called diabetes mellitus (DM). An inadequate supply and/or inadequate effect of insulin causes altered metabolism of carbohydrates, fats, and proteins. This disorder is chronic. The alteration in metabolism may eventually lead to serious complications involving the blood vessels and nerves.

Section 3: INTERVENTIONS TO IMPROVE DIGESTIVE AND METABOLIC FUNCTION

1. Dietary modification:

- Due to acute episodes, the gastrointestinal tract is frequently "put at rest" and nothing is ingested orally (NPO). Placement of nasogastric or intestinal tubes with intermittent suction removes gastric and intestinal secretions. Intravenous administration of fluids and nutrients provides cellular needs.

- Total parenteral nutrition (TPN) or hyperalimentation provides cellular nutrients via intravenous route when oral intake is inadequate or contraindicated. TPN administration includes either or both of the following solutions: amino acid-dextrose solutions or fat emulsions. The amino acid-dextrose solutions contain a hypertonic dextrose solution with additives of sodium, potassium, chloride, calcium, magnesium, phosphate, and trace elements.

— Administration typically occurs through an indwelling subclavian catheter with the insertion site located in the supraclavicular, infraclavicular, antecubital fossa, or internal jugular vein which leads to the superior vena cava.

— The dextrose solutions are hypertonic (20% glucose) and appear clear. Fat emulsions are isotonic and appear white and opaque.

— Persons receiving TPN are susceptible to secondary infections and the underlying debilitated state increases the risk. Hypertonicity of the solution and a long-term indwelling catheter add to the risk. Most institutional policies recommend changing insertion site dressings every 48-72 hours. An additional filter, added to the infusion line, traps bacteria and particles from the dextrose solution.

— Altered serum glucose levels may occur and depend upon the infusion rate. For example, when the infusion rate is faster than the rate of glucose metabolism, hyperglycemia develops which often requires insulin supplementation. Monitoring serum glucose levels every 4-6 hours minimizes adverse serum glucose imbalances.

— Administration requires an infusion pump to minimize flow rate problems. Other intravenous fluids or medications are not administered through TPN delivery lines.

• Varying degrees of altered protein metabolism accompany liver dysfunction. Delayed conversion of ammonia into urea occurs. Limiting the intake of protein to meet only cellular requirements decreases the production of ammonia and urea. Pharmacologic agents provide an alternative for ammonia removal.

— Sufficient energy sources for cellular metabolism require a sufficient daily intake of carbohydrate and calories. If an insufficient caloric intake occurs, the breakdown of tissue protein serves as the energy source. In turn, accumulation of ammonia and urea may develop.

- Obstructed flow of bile from the liver into the duodenum impairs the digestion of ingested fats. Limiting the dietary intake of fatty foods decreases the stimulation and release of bile.

- Varying degrees of altered nutrient digestion accompanies pancreatic dysfunction. Restored pancreatic function requires pharmacologic supplementation.

  — In acute pancreatic dysfunction, diminished flow of pancreatic enzymes into the duodenum occurs. Putting the gastrointestinal tract at rest by providing nothing by mouth (NPO) decreases the stimulation and release of enzymes. Nasogastric intubation with intermittent suction minimizes the accumulation of gastric and intestinal secretions.

  — Altered response to circulating glucose and release of insulin accompany pancreatic dysfunction. Monitoring the clinical manifestations and serum glucose levels provides data for appropriate insulin supplementation.

2. Medication therapy:

- Lactulose (Cephulac) is a complex glucose substance which undergoes a change in the colon forming an acidotic medium. In this environment, ammonia moves from the blood, which circulates in the vessels of the colon wall, into the large intestine. Combined with the osmotic laxative effect of Lactulose, ammonia is rapidly expelled. The routes of administration include oral, nasogastric tube, or retention enema.

- Digestive enzyme replacement provides pancreatic enzymes in the duodenum when dietary substances are also present. These aids facilitate the digestion and absorption of protein, fats and carbohydrates thereby decreasing the nitrogen (ammonia) and fat content in the stool. Examples include pancreatin (Elzyme 303 Enseals), and pancrelipase (Cotazym, Pancrease).

- Insulin supplementation during the management of an acute episode of pancreatitis or DM involves the administration of regular insulin. Regular insulin is the only form that can safely be administered intravenously. Current serum glucose levels determine the dosage. A "sliding scale" of dosage refers to physician orders which determine the dosages of regular insulin appropriate for specific serum glucose levels.

  — Clinical signs of hypoglycemia (excess insulin, insulin shock) include: profuse sweating, headache, nausea, tremors, palpitations, tachycardia, weakness, numbness (especially circumoral), confusion, progressive fatigue, slurred speech, uncontrolled yawning.

3. **Pain control:**

- Severe pain accompanies acute pancreatic inflammatory episodes. Regular administration of nonopiate narcotic analgesics controls the severity of pain without potentiating the spasm of the sphincter of Oddi. Meperidine (Demerol) is the analgesic frequently prescribed. While very effective, it has a hypotensive effect requiring cardiovascular monitoring during the acute phase of treatment and the frequent administration of large dosages.

  — Poorly controlled pain stimulates the vomiting center often producing persistent vomiting despite an essentially empty stomach and duodenum.

  — Intravenous fluid administration replaces losses and restores intravascular volume and perfusion.

A state of shock often accompanies an acute episode. Fluid losses, "third spacing," and neurogenic response to the intense pain accentuate a state of shock.

4. Monitoring systemic response:

- Monitoring of laboratory values assesses trends in hepatic and/or pancreatic dysfunction and healing. Depending upon the laboratory equipment used, the following values are typically within normal parameters.

- Indirect (unconjugated) bilirubin normally is < 0.8 mg/dl. Values increase with hemolysis or rapid destruction of RBC's.

- Direct (conjugated) bilirubin normally is 0.2-0.4 mg/dl. Values increase with hepatic cellular injury or obstructed bile flow.

- Serum albumin normally is 3.5-5.5 gm/dl. Below normal values occur with hepatocellular dysfunction and decreased production of plasma proteins. Increased capillary permeability in the kidneys or in the periphery leads to the loss of albumin from the vascular compartment. Protein and fluid movement into the interstitial space results from capillary permeability.

- Serum amylase normally is 60-180 Somogyi units/ml. Elevated values occur with pancreatic inflammation and obstructed flow of pancreatic enzymes into the duodenum.

- Aspartate amino-transferase (AST), formerly SGOT, normally is 7-40 U/L. Elevated values occur with tissue injury in the liver, heart, kidney, and skeletal muscle.

- Alanine amino-transferase (ALT), formerly SGPT, normally is 7-35 U/L. Elevated values occur with biliary obstruction and injury to the cells lining the biliary tract, bone, intestine, and placenta.

- Blood ammonia levels normally are < 75 ug/100 ml or 9-33 u/mol/L. Elevated values occur with severe hepatocellular damage and contribute to hepatic encephalopathy.

5. **Monitoring for early onset of dysfunction of other body systems:**

   - Renal dysfunction subsequently may develop into impaired perfusion to the kidneys (hepatorenal syndrome). The development of this complication indicates poor prognosis. Some medications such as acetaminophen (Tylenol), indomethacin (Indocin), and aspirin (acetylsalicylic acid) may precipitate renal failure.

   - Hepatic encephalopathy is a complication arising from accumulation of ammonia in the blood. Ammonia acts as a CNS depressant which initially manifests as reduced mental alertness and confusion. This state may progress to loss of consciousness and irreversible coma. Other signs of liver failure accompany hepatic encephalopathy.

   - Pre-existing cardiac conditions may accentuate liver dysfunction. When the right side of the heart is unable to sufficiently pump venous blood through the cardiac chambers, the venous blood backs up into abdominal organs, mainly the liver. The accumulative effects of venous congestion secondary to right-sided heart failure and the portal hypertension may produce an acute episode of hepatic failure.

     — Pre-existing liver dysfunction may also accentuate cardiac dysfunction. An acute episode of liver dysfunction impairs venous return to the heart. Ascites, and an elevated diaphragm with impaired respiratory function and altered gas exchange may diminish the pumping effectiveness of the heart. Progressive heart failure secondary to liver dysfunction may develop.

Section 4: COMMON EXAMPLES OF HIGH ACUITY DIGESTIVE AND METABOLIC CONDITIONS

Diabetes Mellitus (DM)

This chronic condition refers to altered metabolism of carbohydrates, fats, and proteins due to the inadequate supply and/or inadequate effect of insulin. DM is characterized by abnormally high blood (serum) glucose levels (hyperglycemia) and the presence of inadequate metabolism, evidenced by the presence of ketone bodies in the blood and urine.

1. Types of diabetes mellitus:

Type 1: Insulin-dependent diabetes mellitus (IDDM). The pancreas secretes negligible amounts of insulin. The onset typically occurs in childhood or young adulthood.

Type 2: Noninsulin-dependent diabetes mellitus (NIDDM). The pancreas secretes insulin but often in insufficient quantities for the adult body size and activity. An abnormal response to insulin may also result in DM. The onset of NIDDM typically occurs in middle to late adulthood. Obesity is one modifiable risk factor in the development of NIDDM.

- Secondary Diabetes Mellitus. Other pathophysiological conditions precipitate this type of diabetes mellitus. Persons with inadequate functioning pancreatic tissue (pancreatitis, pancreatic cancer) may develop a deficiency in insulin production and subsequently diabetes mellitus. Certain medications produce altered blood glucose levels which require medical management similar to the standard treatment of diabetes mellitus.

- Altered serum glucose levels may develop with the aggressive intervention of another physiological condition. Hypoglycemia may occur with excess alcohol ingestion, high doses of salicylates, or MAO inhibitors. Hyperglycemia may occur with the administration of beta-adrenergic blockers (propranolol), glucocorticoid steroids, nicotinic acid, and some diuretics.

2. **Systemic effects of long-standing or poorly controlled DM:**

- Atherosclerosis develops at an earlier age for persons with DM compared to nondiabetic persons of comparable chronological age. The risk for essential hypertension, acute myocardial infarction, and chronic renal failure is greater for persons with IDDM.

- Peripheral neuropathy develops among persons with long-standing DM. With decreased sensation in feet and toes accompanied by varying degrees of atherosclerosis, the risk for peripheral tissue injury increases. Small tissue injury, such as a blister on the heel from tight fitting shoes, or immobility, may heal poorly and develop into major tissue damage. Amputation of pedal digits or extremities may result.

- Impaired circulation may affect the retina resulting in blindness. Photocoagulation is a laser beam procedure which destroys the abnormal changes in the retinal vessels. This procedure minimizes the occurrence of retinal hemorrhages.

- The development of cataracts and glaucoma occurs more frequently and often at an earlier age among persons with long-standing or poorly controlled DM. Regular eye examinations and assessment of intraocular pressure detect early onset of these conditions. Medications control intraocular pressure and delay the progression of glaucoma which may lead to blindness.

Diabetic Ketoacidosis (DKA)

This potentially life-threatening condition results from insulin deficiency or an inability of the cells to utilize available insulin. A history of Type 1 (IDDM) is common.

Due to prompt intervention and sophisticated monitoring techniques, the estimated mortality rate is 10%.

1. Pathophysiology:

- Tissue cells are unable to obtain glucose molecules from the plasma and glucose is not adequately released from the stores in the liver. The pancreas also increases the release of glucagon which promotes the conversion of stored glycogen to glucose in the liver. These actions produce hyperglycemia and intracellular starvation.

- Plasma hyperglycemia produces osmotic diuresis with an associated loss of sodium in the urine. Dehydration and hypovolemic shock develops. Tissue/cellular metabolism converts to an anaerobic state as tissue ischemia and hypoxia develop. Lactic acidosis progresses to a life-threatening state.

  — ABG's reveal metabolic acidosis with falling pH and HCO_3 values.

  — Potassium and hydrogen molecules exchange across the cell wall in an attempt to compensate for the acidotic state. The cells take in hydrogen in exchange for the release of potassium. The kidneys normally filter and remove the excess potassium. With normal function, serum potassium values remain within normal range. However, if renal failure develops (due to poor perfusion and hypovolemia), serum potassium values may reach seriously elevated levels. Cardiac ventricular dysrhythmias may occur.

- When cells are unable to use glucose for energy and metabolic activity, the body breaks down tissue protein and body fat to produce energy for cellular functions. Fat breakdown results in the accumulation of ketone bodies which leads to ketoacidosis. The acidotic state worsens.

- As the state of metabolic acidosis progresses, the serum pH decreases and the functioning of other body systems decreases. Depression of the respiratory and neurological systems occurs which leads to coma and respiratory failure.

2. Indications:

The onset, typically, is slow with gradual progression of symptoms. Precipitating factors include psychological, emotional, or physical stressors such as surgery, trauma, pregnancy, and insufficient insulin administration. Inadequate insulin administration or inappropriate dietary intake accounts for the majority of acute episodes of DKA.

- Classic signs of DKA include: polyuria; polydipsia; polyphagia; weight loss. Other signs of an acute episode of DKA include: fatigue/lethargy; nausea and vomiting; abdominal pain.

- Signs associated with dehydration include: dry, flushed skin; dry mucous membrane; poor skin turgor; hypotension; tachycardia.

- Signs associated with acidosis and accumulated ketone bodies include: decreased LOC (lethargy or coma); deep and rapid respirations (Kussmaul); fruity odor to the breath.

- Although the values may vary according to the laboratory equipment used, the following parameters are typical of diagnostic tests for adults experiencing an acute episode of DKA.

  — Serum glucose: 200-800 mg/dl

  — Serum ketones: elevated

  — Urine glucose: positive

  — Urine acetone (ketone bodies): positive

  — Serum osmolality: 300-350 mOsm/L

  — Serum pH: 7.30

Focused Bedside Assessment

The following is a guideline of expected data from a head-to-toe assessment of an adult experiencing an acute episode of diabetic ketoacidosis (DKA) and the associated body system involved. Pathophysiological problems not related to DKA and the systemic effects are not included.

- **General Appearance:** lethargic, stupor or coma; flushed appearance; weakness; dry skin; poor skin turgor ("tenting").

- **Neurological Status:** decreased LOC with slow response and poor orientation; pupils dilated and react equally to light. Other concurrent neurological problems include history of TIA or CVA.

- **Cardiac/Circulatory Status:** blood pressure below person's normal parameters (may be hypotensive), tachycardia; perhaps PVC's if potassium imbalance is present. Other concurrent cardiac problems include hypertension, history of MI, CHF, or heart block dysrhythmias.

- **Respiratory Status:** Kussmaul's respirations (deep and rapid); acetone (sweet) odor to breath; lung sounds may be congested. Other concurrent respiratory problems include COPD or asthma.

- **Abdominal Status:** nausea and vomiting; abdominal pain and rigidity; diminished bowel sounds; dry mucous membranes.

- **Urinary Elimination Status:** initially may exhibit polyuria and later develop oliguria if shock is present; protein, sugar, and ketone present in urine.

- **Extremities:** weakness; paresthesia; weak peripheral pulses, especially if shock state is present.

- When the individual is turned to his/her side, the nurse would expect to find dry, flushed skin; poor skin turgor.

If additional data are observed, a more detailed assessment of the involved body system is required. Additional areas of physiological dysfunction may be present and confound the present metabolic problem.

— Serum sodium: 135 mEq/L

— Serum potassium: normal or elevated 5.5 mEq/L

— ABG: metabolic acidosis; sometimes combined respiratory and metabolic acidosis

3. Medical and Nursing Management (for an adult):

• Rehydration to correct dehydration is essential to minimize adverse effects on other body systems. The administration of IV fluids (normal saline or 0.45% saline) restores a normovolemic or hemodynamically stable state as evidenced by:

— Blood pressure: 110/70 mmHg or the person's normal range

— Heart rate: 60-100 bpm

— CVP: 2-6 mmHg

— PAWP (PCOP): 6-12 mmHg

— Urinary output: ≥ 30 ml/hr

• Continuous administration of rapid-acting insulin via intravenous route progressively lowers the serum glucose level. With the utilization of insulin, the severity of the ketoacidosis decreases. The state of metabolic acidosis improves as is evidenced by the gradual rise in the pH and HCO_3 values.

— Initial or loading doses of regular insulin typically are 10-25 units or 0.3 U/Kg of body weight. The dosage for continuous infusion is typically 5-10 units per hour or 0.1 U/Kg/hr. Frequent monitoring of the serum glucose levels determines dosage adjustments. Rapid decrease in serum glucose levels minimizes the precipitation of hypoglycemia and electrolyte imbalances.

• Identification of the cause of ketoacidosis is essential. Respiratory or urinary tract infections are the most common precipitating cause. Subacute vaginal and urinary tract infections may also be present.

Cultures of respiratory secretions and urine determine the presence of pathogens. Obtaining cultures precedes the initiation of antibiotic therapy.

— Long-standing protein depletion increases the susceptibility to infections. Good skin care, meticulous handwashing, and aseptic care of invasive monitoring sites minimize the development of nosocomial infections.

• Replacement of electrolytes are in accordance with serum values. IV fluid administration restores fluid deficit and sodium losses.

— Monitoring serum potassium while correcting dehydration and acidosis minimize iatrogenic complications. As the serum pH rises, hydrogen moves out of the cells and potassium returns to the intracellular compartment. Hypokalemia may result and require potassium replacement. (Refer to Unit 6 for additional information on the treatment of potassium imbalance.)

• The insertion of a nasogastric tube during the early treatment period minimizes the occurrence of aspiration from vomitus especially if coma is also present. When severe and acute acidosis occurs, the body attempts to lower systemic sources of hydrogen by eliminating acidotic gastric secretions through vomiting. With decreased LOC, aspiration of emesis may occur. Subsequent pneumonitis may lead to ARDS and respiratory failure.

Hyperosmolar, Hypertonic Nonketotic Coma (HHNC)

This life-threatening emergency results from insulin deficiency characterized by severe elevation of the blood glucose, profound dehydration, and decreased level of consciousness. An absence of ketone bodies differentiates this condition from diabetic ketoacidosis. Typically, the person with HHNC is elderly with Type 2 (NIDDM) diabetes mellitus and a concurrent infection despite aggressive treatment and sophisticated monitoring techniques. The estimated mortality rate is 20-50%.

1. Pathophysiology:

- Persons with severe hyperglycemia also have severe hyperglysuria. Body water moves to the location of excess glucose, therefore, the kidneys excrete large volumes of water producing a state of progressive and profound dehydration. Persons may lose 25% of their total body water.

- Rapidly developing dehydration occurs. Renal blood flow decreases leading to renal ischemia and impaired renal function. Acute tubular necrosis (ATN) and acute renal failure (ARF) may result.

- As the intravascular volume decreases, the blood becomes viscid and flow slows. As this state of hemoconcentration progresses, platelet aggregation and adhesiveness increases. The risk of thrombus and emboli increases. Cerebral vascular accident, pulmonary emboli, and renal infarction may result from intravascular clot formation or decreased perfusion.

- A sequence of intravascular, interstitial and intracellular fluid depletion develops. Intracellular dehydration causes cells to shrink. Neurological deficits develop but may be difficult to recognize as the symptoms of the onset are gradual and insidious among an elderly population.

2. Indications:

- The typical person with HHNC is over 50 years of age with a preexisting cardiac or pulmonary condition. A relatively minor respiratory or urinary tract infection may precipitate the complications.

  — As elderly persons have delayed onset of the physical signs of infection and normally have subnormal body temperatures, the increased metabolic needs and elevated body temperature associated with an infection are often unnoticed and undetected. The WBC value is typically elevated despite normal body temperature.

- Ketone bodies are not usually present in the serum or urine. A state of acidosis occurs secondary to dehydration. The degree of acidosis is typically less severe than that of DKA.

- Serum glucose levels are typically greater than 600 mg/dL and may be as high as 2000 mg/dl. The serum osmolality is typically greater than 350 mOsm/L. Due to prolonged osmotic diuresis, the degree of dehydration is typically more severe compared to DKA.

  — Due to intravascular depletion, impaired perfusion to the kidneys results. Renal ischemia and acute tubular necrosis (ATN) often develop as reflected by elevated BUN and serum creatinine levels.

  — As the vascular volume decreases and blood components become concentrated, the hematocrit elevates. Platelets aggregate and adhere forming thrombi and emboli. Secondary CVA and PE frequently develop.

- Decreased LOC with associated cerebral edema occurs. Glucose and associated water molecules freely move across the blood-brain barrier. While this phenomenon ensures an adequate nutritional supply for brain activity, it may complicate the treatment measures.

- Metabolic acidosis is less severe compared to DKA because of the minimal presence of ketone bodies with HHNC.

3. Medical and Nursing Management:

- Administration of hypotonic IV solutions (0.45% saline) corrects dehydration and hyperosmolar serum. As much as 8-10 liters of fluid may be required during the first 8-10 hours of treatment.

  — A risk for overcorrecting the dehydration and subsequently precipitating pulmonary edema exists. Therefore, close monitoring of cardiac and circulatory status is essential. Shifts in serum electrolytes (potassium and sodium) occur with the correction of dehydration.

- .Administration of rapid acting insulin is gradual for a steady lowering of the serum glucose level. Avoiding high doses of insulin and rapid serum glucose reduction are essential since the risk for increasing cerebral edema is high.

  — The relationship of glucose and body fluid movement across the blood-brain barrier underlies the risk of cerebral edema. With HHNC, the blood-brain barrier permits the movement of large quantities of glucose into brain tissue. If the serum level is lowered faster than the movement of glucose from the brain tissue back into the vascular space, greater glucose levels remain in the brain tissue. To accompany the elevated glucose levels, water molecules move from the vascular space into the brain tissue to accompany the elevated glucose levels. The risk for cerebral edema and dangerously impaired cerebral perfusion pressures increases. Gradual lowering of serum glucose and subsequently glucose levels in brain tissue minimizes the risk of evolving cerebral edema.

- Hemodynamic monitoring is essential to assess the benefits and effects of fluid replacement. Pre-existing cardiac and pulmonary conditions often complicate a plan for aggressive restoration of fluid volume.

Hepatic Failure

Hepatic failure refers to the loss of liver function because of extensive cellular damage. The damage may develop slowly as with cirrhosis or suddenly as with acute hepatitis. Approximately 80% of the liver is nonfunctional before symptoms appear. Hepatic tissue has regenerative capability; however, liver failure refers to less than 15% of functioning liver capacity.

1. Pathophysiology:

- Cirrhosis is a chronic liver disease associated with widespread tissue necrosis and irreversible fibrotic changes within the liver. Common causes include chronic alcohol ingestion, recurrent viral hepatitis, and metabolic disorders.

- Sudden and severe liver decompensation with massive cellular necrosis characterize acute hepatic failure. Common causes include hepatitis, drug reactions, poisoning, or systemic shock.

- The failing liver is unable to metabolize bilirubin resulting in jaundice. The risk of asterixis (brain damage) increases.

- Inadequate protein metabolism results in an accumulation of ammonia in the blood which produces neurological toxicity (hepatic encephalopathy). The liver no longer is able to convert ammonia to urea for elimination.

- Diminished blood flow through the liver leads to vascular congestion (portal hypertension). Congestion in the intestinal circulation leads to ascites, esophageal varices, and hemorrhoids. Decreased venous return to the right side of the heart contributes to impaired pulmonary circulation and altered gas exchange. In turn, decreased blood flow through the left side of the heart leads to diminished systemic perfusion. Reduction in renal perfusion leads to renal failure secondary to hepatic dysfunction (hepatorenal syndrome).

- Inadequate vitamin K absorption leads to bleeding tendencies. The liver progressively is unable to synthesize clotting factors.

2. Indications:

- Jaundice results from inadequate bilirubin metabolism and accumulation in the systemic circulation. It is particularly noticeable in the unexposed skin, sclera and mucous membranes.

  — Dark-colored urine is due to bilirubin. This symptom is apparent several days prior to the onset of jaundice.

  — Pale-colored stool is due to the absence of bilirubin in intestinal contents.

- Weight gain is due to fluid retention. Peripheral edema and ascites contribute to weight gain. Skeletal muscle wasting is present.

3. Medical and Nursing Management:

- Correcting the precipitating factor is essential for delaying the progression of cellular damage.

- Abnormal fluid and electrolyte values require correction.

  — Unless hyponatremia is profound, dietary sodium is restricted to minimize ascites, peripheral edema, and renal insufficiency.

  — Fresh frozen plasma is used for blood replacements as it contains clotting factors. Albumin is used with fluid resuscitation to restore oncotic pressure and intravascular volume. CVP and PAP monitoring are essential to ensure adequate tissue perfusion without fluid overload.

Focused Bedside Assessment

The following is a guideline of expected data from a head-to-toe assessment of an adult experiencing hepatic failure and the associated body system involvement. Pathophysiological problems not related to hepatic failure and the systemic effects are not included.

- **General Appearance:** jaundice; emaciated with skeletal muscle atrophy; scant body hair distribution; head hair is thin and dry; malaise and weakness; lethargy.

- **Neurological Status:** poor memory, drowsy; pupils equal and react to light.

- **Cardiac/Circulatory Status:** normal to bounding pulses; low to normal blood pressure; elevated cardiac output when decreased peripheral resistance occurs. Impaired right ventricular filling leads to decreased circulation through the heart. At risk for septic shock and variceal hemorrhage.

- **Respiratory Status:** may have basal congestion; labored breathing due to elevated diaphragm; prefers Fowler's position for easier breathing. Breast tissue enlargement on males (gynecomastia). Spider angiomas which blanch with digital pressure on trunk and abdomen.

- **Abdominal Status:** profound distention due to ascites; noticeable cutaneous vessels especially around the umbilicus. Liver may be enlarged and tender or hard and nodular. Ecchymoses on body surfaces. Foul-smelling breath especially if stomatitis present. Dullness percussed over the fluid accumulation.

- **Urinary Elimination Status:** urinary output dependent upon fluid status; testicular atrophy or amenorrhea.

- **Extremities:** peripheral edema of lower extremities; ecchymoses; palmar erythema.

- When the individual is turned to his/her side, the nurse would expect to find: Ecchymoses; sacral edema.

If additional data are observed, a more detailed assessment of the involved body system is required. Additional areas of pathophysiological dysfunction may be present and confound the present hepatic problem.

- Decreased physical activity or bedrest conserves metabolic requirements. A high calorie and high protein diet provides optimal supply of nutrients unless encephalopathy is present. Supplemental parenteral nutrition provides caloric needs when dietary intake is inadequate. High calorie intake minimizes the utilization of tissue protein to meet cellular metabolic needs. Glucose intake counterbalances the potential for hypoglycemia which frequently occurs when gluconeogenesis is inadequate.

- Histamine H_2-receptor antagonists, such as cimetidine (Tagamet) and ranitidine (Zantac), minimize the development of gastric ulceration.

- The management of symptoms of hepatic encephalopathy includes decreasing protein intake and administering enemas to remove intestinal contents and ammonia producing bacteria. Oral neomycin, a nonabsorbable antibiotic, reduces intestinal bacteria in acute situations. Lactulose, a disaccharide, facilitates the elimination of ammonia through the large intestine.

- A surgically placed shunt system, such as portocaval, splenorenal, mesocaval shunt provides vascular bypass to minimize the backup of blood or severe hypertension within the portal system.

  — The LeVeen procedure provides continual removal of fluids for persons with life-threatening ascites. This surgical procedure drains accumulated peritoneal fluid by means of a long subcutaneous catheter placed between the abdomen and the superior vena cava. A pressure-sensitive valve regulates the fluid flow.

- Persons with irreversible, progressive liver disease who have minimal dysfunction of other body systems are possible candidates for hepatic transplantation.

Bleeding Esophageal Varices

When the portal venous pressure increases above normal parameters of 7 mmHg to 20-25 mmHg, small vessels surrounding the lower esophagus and stomach become distended. Sudden increases in vascular pressure or mechanical irritation cause these thin-walled engorged vessels to bleed. Thrombocytopenia and clotting disorders accentuate the risk of blood loss.

1. Indications:

- Sudden and dramatic onset of bleeding produces hematemesis of bright red blood and blood clots. When blood mixes with gastric secretions, it becomes black. Small amounts of blood mixed with gastric secretions produce a "coffee ground" appearance to the emesis. Blood that passes through the intestinal tract produces black, tarry stools or diarrhea. Melena refers to blood in the stool.

  — Several units of blood may be lost during a single bleeding episode. Due to the severity of blood loss, hypovolemic shock rapidly develops.

  — Occasionally, persons experiencing minor bleeding perceive an accompanying sense of doom or feeling that something serious is about to happen. Prompt examination and identification of the bleeding site prevent major blood loss.

2. Medical and Nursing Management:

- With minor bleeding, an esophagoscopy visualizes the varices and bleeding site. The injection of varices with a sclerosing solution, such as sodium tetradecyl sulphate, produces obliteration and fibrosis. The recurrence of bleeding episodes decreases.

- The inflation of esophageal and gastric balloons which surround the multiple lumen nasogastric tube temporarily controls acute bleeding. A Sengstaken-Blakemore or similar multiple lumen tube achieves a

Blakemore-Sengstaken Tube

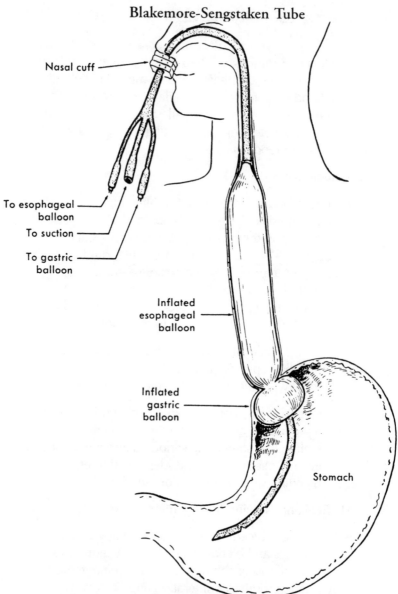

Nasal cuff

To esophageal balloon

To suction

To gastric balloon

Inflated esophageal balloon

Inflated gastric balloon

Stomach

Barbara Long, Wilma Phipps, Essentials of Medical Surgical Nursing: A Nursing Process Approach, Saint Louis: Mosby-Year Book, 1991. Reprinted by permission of Mosby-Year Book and Davol, Inc. Providence, Rhode Island) tamponade pressure on bleeding sites. The tube is secured with some external tension to a football-type helmet with a face guard.

— One lumen permits the inflation of an esophageal balloon. A second lumen permits the inflation of an upper gastric balloon.

— Intermittent suction aspirates blood and clots through a third lumen. Lavage with saline through this lumen removes blood from the stomach.

— Removal of blood is essential because excessive breakdown of RBC's during hemorrhage produces increased quantities of unconjugated bilirubin. The amount of bilirubin typically exceeds the ability of the liver to convert it to water-soluble form for urinary elimination (hemolytic jaundice).

Pancreatitis

An inflammation of the pancreas may be acute or chronic. The acute form presents dramatic symptoms and a high mortality rate because of widespread necrosis and hemorrhage.

1. Pathophysiology:

• Initially, the pancreatic ducts become obstructed causing injury to adjacent cells where inactive pancreatic enzymes are stored. The damaged cells release stored enzymes into the pancreatic tissue which surrounds the damaged area. Reflux of duodenal contents and bile back into the pancreatic ducts further activates this autodigestive response.

• Ingested food and gastric secretions stimulate the release of additional pancreatic enzymes which are unable to flow into the duodenum. The secondary inflammatory response and localized edema leads to further occlusion, of the duct system within the pancreas. A cycle of accumulating activated enzymes, inflammation, progressive duct occlusion, and tissue erosion evolves.

— Expanding inflammation leads to obstructed blood flow to pancreatic tissue. Tissue ischemia progresses to tissue necrosis and abscess formation.

— Expanding erosion of pancreatic tissue leads to damage of the vessels within the pancreas. Varying degrees of intrapancreatic bleeding occur.

• Edema and vascular injury frequently lead to rupture of pancreatic ducts and spillage of enzyme secretions into the peritoneal cavity. Chemical peritonitis results.

2. **Indications:**

• Persistent and frequentl severe abdominal pain occurs suddenly and typically following excessive food or alcohol intake. The location of the pain is often mid-epigastric radiating to the right upper quadrant or through to the back.

• Accompanying gastrointestinal symptoms include: nausea and vomiting; diarrhea; melena; hematemesis; diminished bowel sounds.

• Other systemic symptoms reflect the degree of sepsis and hemorrhagic shock involvement. (Refer to Unit 4 for the indications of shock.)

• Typical laboratory findings (which may vary according to the laboratory equipment used) include:

— Elevated serum amylase (> 180 SI units/ml) indicates pancreatic inflammation and obstructed enzyme flow.

— Decreased serum albumin (< 3.5 g/dl) indicates interstitial fluid retention.

— Decreased serum calcium (< 8 mg/dl). Calcium is protein bound, therefore hypocalcemia accompanies a low serum albumin level. If not promptly identified and treated, hypocalcemia may precipitate cardiac ventricular dysrhythmias.

— Elevated WBC indicates an inflammatory response.

— Elevated serum glucose (> 200 mg/dl) indicates inadequate release of insulin.

— Decreased platelet and fibrinogen levels with elevated fibrin levels contribute to the bleeding and development of microthrombi.

3. **Medical and Nursing Management:**

- Interventions focus on pain relief, fluid replacement, and minimal stimulation of pancreatic activity until the autodigestion subsides.

  — Meperidine (Demerol) provides optimal pain relief compared to Morphine which often produces spasms of the smooth muscles of the pancreatic ducts and ampulla of Vater.

  — As the inflammatory process produces fluid movement from the intravascular space, fluid resuscitation minimizes the degree of hypovolemic shock. Colloidal fluids, albumin, and fresh frozen plasma replace vascular losses. Monitored electrolyte values determine replacement.

  — Withholding all oral intake and aspiration of gastric secretions decrease gastrointestinal activity and in turn decrease the stimulation of pancreatic enzyme excretion. Parenteral feedings provide nutritional support during the acute phase.

- Respiratory insufficiency may develop due to inadequate ventilation which develops as a secondary response to the intensity of the upper abdominal pain and inadequate circulatory perfusion. Monitoring oxygen saturation provides early data on the development of pulmonary congestion, pleural effusion and atelectasis. Respiratory failure may develop. (Refer to Unit 2 for additional information of respiratory failure.)

Focused Bedside Assessment

The following is a guideline of expected data from a head-to-toe assessment of an adult experiencing an acute episode of pancreatitis and the associated body system involvement. Pathophysiological problems not related to acute pancreatitis and the systemic effects are not included.

- **General Appearance:** sudden onset of acute epigastric or umbilical pain apparent; flexed body position; fever; pallor; jaundice may be present.

- **Neurological Status:** initially hyperalert and focused on severity of pain; pupils equal, round, and reactive to light accommodation.

- **Cardiac/Circulatory Status:** clinical signs of shock (hypotension, tachycardia, and poor peripheral perfusion); PVC's may develop.

- **Respiratory Status:** congested lung sounds due to pleural effusion; may exhibit pain with breathing indicating pleural involvement. Rapid often shallow respirations due to pain. At risk for developing ARDS.

- **Abdominal Status:** persistent vomiting; abdominal distention, firm with upper to middle quadrant pain; diminished bowel sounds in lower abdomen.

- **Extremities:** no unusual findings; feet may be cool with diminished peripheral pulses if shock is present.

- When the individual is turned to his/her side, the nurse would expect to find: no unusual or specific findings.

If additional data are observed, a more detailed assessment of the involved body system is required. Additional areas of physiological dysfunction may be present and confound the present pancreatic problem.

Appendix A

List of NANDA Nursing Diagnoses

* Activity Intolerance
* Activity Intolerance, Risk for
* Adaptive Capacity, Decreased Intracranial
* Adjustment, Impaired
* Airway Clearance, Ineffective
* Anxiety
* Aspiration, Risk for
* Body Image Disturbance
* Body Temperature, Risk for Altered
* Breastfeeding, Effective
* Breastfeeding, Ineffective
* Breastfeeding, Interrupted
* Breathing Pattern, Ineffective
* Cardiac Output, Decreased
* Caregiver Role Strain
* Communications, Impaired Verbal
* Community Coping, Ineffective
* Community Coping, Potential for Enhanced
* Confusion, Acute
* Confusion, Chronic
* Constipation
* Constipation, Colonic

* Constipation, Perceived

* Coping, Ineffective Individual

* Decisional Conflict (Specify)

* Denial, Ineffective

* Diarrhea

* Disuse Syndrome, Risk for

* Diversional Activity Deficit

* Dysfunctional Ventilatory Weaning Response

* Dysreflexia

* Energy Field, Disturbance

* Environmental Interpretation Syndrome, Impaired

* Family Coping, Compromised, Ineffective

* Family Coping, Disabling, Ineffective

* Family Coping, Potential for Growth

* Family Processes, Altered

* Family Processes, Altered, Alcoholism

* Fatigue

* Fear

* Fluid Volume Deficit

* Fluid Volume Deficit, Risk for

* Fluid Volume Excess

* Gas Exchange, Impaired

* Grieving, Anticipatory

* Grieving, Dysfunctional

* Growth and Development, Altered

* Health Maintenance, Altered

* Health-seeking Behaviors (Specify)

* Home Maintenance Management, Impaired

* Hopelessness

* Hyperthermia

* Hypothermia

* Incontinence, Bowel

* Incontinence, Functional

* Incontinence, Reflex

* Incontinence, Stress

* Incontinence, Total

* Incontinence, Urge

* Infant Behavior, Disorganized

* Infant Behavior, Potential for Enhanced Organized

* Infant Behavior, Risk for Disorganized

* Infant Feeding Pattern, Ineffective

* Infection, Risk for

* Injury, Risk for

* Knowledge Deficit (Specify)

* Loneliness, Risk for

* Management of Therapeutic Regimen, Effective, Individual

* Management of Therapeutic Regimen, Ineffective Community

* Management of Therapeutic Regimen, Ineffective Family

* Memory, Impaired

* Noncompliance (Specify)

* Nutrition: Less than Body Requirements, Altered

* Nutrition: More the Body Requirements, Altered

* Oral Mucous Membrane. Altered

* Pain

* Pain, Chronic

* Parent/Infant/Child Attachment, Risk for Altered

* Parental Role Conflict

* Parenting, Altered

* Parenting, Risk for Altered

* Perioperative Positioning, Risk for Injury

* Peripheral Neurovascular Dysfunction, Risk for

* Personal Identity Disturbance

* Physical Mobility, Impaired

* Poisoning, Risk for

* Post-Trauma Responses

* Powerlessness

* Protection, Altered

* Rape-Trauma Syndrome

* Rape-Trauma Syndrome, Compound Reaction

* Rape-Trauma Syndrome, Silent Reaction

* Relocation Stress Syndrome

* Role Performance, Altered

* Self-Care Deficit, Bathing/Hygiene, Dressing/Grooming, Feeding, Toileting

* Self-Esteem, Chronic Low

* Self-Esteem, Situational Low

* Self-Esteem Disturbance

* Self Mutilation, Risk for

* Sensory/Perceptual Alterations (Specify: visual, auditory, kinesthetic, gustatory, tactile, olfactory)

* Sexual Dysfunction

* Sexual Patterns, Altered

* Skin Integrity, Impaired

* Skin Integrity, Risk for

* Sleep Pattern Disturbance

* Social Interaction, Impaired

* Social Isolation

* Spiritual Distress (Distress of the Human Spirit)

* Spiritual Well Being, Potential for Enhanced

* Suffocation, High Risk for

* Swallowing, Impaired

* Thermoregulation, Ineffective

* Thought Processes, Altered

* Tissue Integrity, Impaired

* Tissue Perfusion, Altered (Specify: renal, cerebral, cardiopulmonary, gastrointestinal, peripheral)

* Tissue Perfusion, Altered Cardiac

* Trauma, Risk for

* Unilateral Neglect

* Urinary Elimination, Altered

* Urinary Retention

* Ventilation, Inability to Sustain Spontaneous

* Violence, Risk for: Self-Directed or Directed to Others

Appendix B

Common Serum Lab Values

Stated values may vary somewhat due to calibration of laboratory equipment. Normal values are typically stated along with patient values for comparison.

Alanine aminotransferase (ALT, SGPT)
    evaluation of liver injury
    0-35 IU/L

Albumin
    major component of plasma protein; essential in maintaining intravascular volume
    3.4-4.7 mg/dL

Alkaline phosphatase
    found in liver, bone, intestine, and placenta
    41-133 IU/L

Ammonia (NH4)
    results from protein metabolism; accumulations toxic to brain tissue
    18-60 ug/dL

Aspartate aminotransferase (AST, SGOT, GOT)
    released with tissue damage (liver, skeletal muscle, brain, RBC, and heart)
    0-35 IU/L

Bilirubin
    elevated with liver disease, biliary obstruction, or hemolysis
    0.1-1.2 mg/dL

Blood urea nitrogen (BUN)
    urea is end product of protein metabolism & normally excreted from the kidneys
    8-20 mg/dL

Calcium
    required for cellular neurotransmission & bone

stability
8.5-10.5 mg/dL

Carbon dioxide (CO_2) total
measurement of circulating bicarbonate ions or estimate of acid-base status
22-28 mEq/L

Chloride
maintains normal acid-base balance
98-107 mEq/L

Clotting time, activated (ACT)
bedside assessment of heparinization
114-186 seconds

Creatine kinase (CK)
released with tissue damage (skeletal muscle,
myocardium, brain)
32-267 IU/L

Creatine kinase MB
specific isoenzyme associated with myocardial damage
< 16 IU/L

Creatinine
end product of metabolism that is excreted with normal renal function
0.6-1.2 mg/dL

Ferritin
estimate of total body stores of iron
females: 4-161 ng/mL   males: 16-300 ng/mL

Glucose
extracellular ion available for cellular energy
60-115 mg/dL

Glucose tolerance test (GTT)
determines the body's ability to respond appropriately
to glucose levels
fasting (< 115 mg/dL), 1hr (< 200 mg/dL), 2hr
(< 140 mg/dL)

Iron-binding capacity, total (TIBC)
250-460 ug/dL

Magnesium
intracellular ion necessary for cellular function
1.8-3.0 mg/dL

Osmolality (serum)
measures osmotic pressure & ability to preserve intracellular & extracellular fluid
285-293 mOsm/Kg

Partial thromboplastin time (PTT)
assessment of response to heparin therapy
25-35 seconds

Potassium
intracellular ion; excess excreted from kidneys
3.5-5.0 mEq/L

Prothrombin time (PT)
assessment of response to Warfarin (Coumadin) therapy
11-15 seconds

Sodium
extracellular ion; related to fluid balance
135-145 mEq/L

Uric acid
end product of protein metabolism & excreted by
kidneys
females: 1.4-5.8 mg/dL   males: 2.4-7.4 mg/dL

Index